At The Bedside

Stories from a career in Emergency Medicine

Mark J. Thomson, M.D.

At The Bedside

First Edition

Copyright c 2022 Mark J. Thomson, M.D.

ISBN: 978-1-387-65975-3

This book is dedicated to my parents,

John and Theresa Thomson

Table of Contents

Introduction

All these stories are true. Personal identification such as names, age, sex, and certain details such as time, location, etc. have been changed so that no patient can be identified. The names of physicians and nurses may or may not have been changed. Over 36 years of practicing emergency medicine I saw approximately 120,000 patients. This book was written from memory. I kept no notes, recordings, or pictures. I did not review any medical records. I am certain many events have blended together. That is how my memory seems to work. The chapters run chronologically. Quotations are recollections of words spoken and are as close to what was actually said as possible.

I studied at Kalamazoo College from 1972 to 1976, and the University of Michigan medical school from 1976 to 1980. I completed a family practice residency program at Providence Hospital in Southfield, Michigan from 1980 to 1983. I began to moonlight in a small "Freestanding" Emergency Department (no attached hospital) in Novi, Michigan in January of 1982. Novi was a small town with a large rural area nearby in the 1980's. It gradually became a large suburban community over the next 36 years. I covered the 12-hour Wednesday night shift for a year and a half. I began my full-time career on July 1st of 1983. During the last ten years of my career, I worked 75 % of my shifts in the Novi ER and 25 % of my shifts in the ER at Allegiance Health Hospital in Jackson, Michigan. Jackson is a medium-sized city, the largest in Jackson County.

Emergency Medicine was first recognized in 1979 by the ABEM (American Board of Emergency Medicine) and was fully approved as a specialty in 1989. In the 1970's - 80's the ED (Emergency Department) was called the ER (Emergency Room), I have kept that designation.

The practice of emergency medicine has many challenging moments. There are a few wonderful "Saves" but many horrible and tragic disasters as well. Putting the triumphs and defeats on paper has added needed perspective to my career. I hope these stories illustrate the character and spirit of ordinary people at significant moments in their lives (of patients and health care providers). I can't describe vividly enough the dramatic feelings and emotions that occur when seeing patients and families at critical times in the ER. To be at the bedside, to participate was the most important thing. Emergency physicians attend patients during serious illness or injury, often life changing events. The work is difficult, at times overwhelming. The famous line from the movie A League of Their Own "It's the hard that makes it great," absolutely applies.

Many of us have seen the quote "Crisis Doesn't Create Character - It Reveals It." I believe that to be true, having seen it many times. Most people are not expecting or prepared for a serious medical emergency. In the anxiety and chaos of a sudden critical illness or significant injury one's moral qualities are often exposed.

In the introduction of the textbook *Harrison's Principles of Internal Medicine* the authors describe what it means to become a physician: "No greater opportunity, responsibility or obligation can fall to a human being than to become a physician. In the care of the suffering one needs technical skill, scientific knowledge, and human understanding. Those who use these with courage, humility and wisdom will provide a unique service for their fellow man; and will build character within themselves." (Ref. 1). I hope this to be true as well.

As I neared completion of writing these stories, I realized many of them involved children. Their tragic cases affected me the most. There is death and dying in the ER. Most cases involve the elderly, fortunately very few involve infants and children. The death of a geriatric patient was sad and occasionally devastating to remaining family and friends. But usually not tragic, as most had completed their life's journey.

There were deaths among young adults: from horribly accidents, drug overdose, suicide, etc. These were difficult to adjust to as well. Many were due to risky behavior: drug wars, guns, knives, and drunk driving (especially on hot summer weekends). While also tragic, these deaths don't leave as deep a scar.

I am older now. My hands tremble a bit. I have seen enough bad outcomes. I worry more. I have left the practice of emergency medicine in the ER to my talented younger colleagues. Four years have passed since my retirement. Long enough (I hope) to process all that has happened.

I need to thank my family. Full time emergency physicians work multiple midnight shifts and 50 percent of all weekends and holidays. I missed many family events. It is one of the few regrets I have about choosing a career in EM.

I want to thank my editors: Natalie Dominguez, John Houle, Lisa Mullenneaux and Jennifer Lamberts. Their insightful suggestions helped me improve and clarify every chapter. Any errors or omissions are my responsibility.

Diener

Good fortune brought me the diener (pathologist assistant) position. My older brothers Tom and Steve held the job previously. It was a springtime assignment for a Kalamazoo College student. I applied the previous fall and had been assured the job. However, three weeks before starting I was notified there was going to be an interview. The pre-med program had decided to reserve the diener position for a pre-med student. My major was biochemistry. A second job was available, at the Kalamazoo city water treatment plant. There was one other student applicant. One of us would get the diener position, the other would work at the water treatment plant. I'd heard about that job. It entailed performing various tests on water samples: checking the turbidity, chlorine concentration and e coli bacteria levels. These biochemistry tests required an hour to carry out, then needed to be repeated every two hours. I talked to a student who'd previously held the position. He said it was interesting the first day, followed by total mind-numbing boredom for weeks.

The interview day arrived. I sat in the reception area next to the other applicant Walter Knight. It was not looking good for me. Walter was polite, poised, and soft spoken. He was a talented and diligent student, one of the top pre-med students at the college. Walter was also a superb tennis player, with picture perfect strokes. He was called into the interview room first. About 20 minutes later he emerged relaxed and smiling. It was my turn. I walked in hesitantly. There were three professors on the interview committee. They began enthusiastically describing the opportunity at the water treatment plant. They asked about my interest in that position. I was livid. They didn't even mention the pathologist's assistant position. I could hardly think of what to say, then blurted out "I'm not sure what's going to happen, but I had been promised the deiner job. You can assign me to the water treatment plant, but I will not show up. On day one, I'm heading to Bronson Hospital." They leaned back, pausing in silence, frowning. I couldn't recall a time I ever spoke so directly to professors. The interview ended quickly. A week later, I was called to the Science Administration Office. The administrative assistant let me know the committee was upset with my attitude and outspoken demeanor. But, they granted my request. Walter was assigned to the water treatment plant. I was awarded the diener position.

———————————

On my first day Dave Kennel (the diener I was replacing) was showing me the duties involved. We started at 7 AM in the hospital laboratory and picked up a phlebotomist tray with equipment to draw blood. We spent an hour taking samples from various patients admitted to the hospital wards, then went downstairs to the autopsy room. There was one case for the day. A deceased elderly male was on the steel autopsy table, covered by a thin white sheet. The body was cold and stiff from rigor mortis. Mottled purplish discoloration was visible along the back, a condition called dependent lividity. I'd only seen two dead bodies in my life, both in caskets at funerals.

Dave reviewed the patient chart and checked the ID tag on the left great toe, they matched. He demonstrated how to gather and spread out the necessary tools: knives, forceps, bone saw, retractors, etc. Shortly after, Dr. Rusher the pathologist arrived. We donned large aprons and gloves. They stepped forward to begin the autopsy. Unsure of myself and feeling a bit lightheaded and nauseated, I held back. I was hoping not to pass out.

The pathologist looked up and said, "You're the new diener?"

"Yes," I nodded.

He motioned me forward and handed me a scalpel. "Follow my lead. We'll do the gross dissection together." Taking a scalpel, he swiftly made a large deep Y incision over the anterior chest and then carried it down the middle of the abdomen. Using a bone saw with an oscillating blade he cut through the right ribs. He handed the saw across to me, I cut through the left ribs. With sharp instruments and blunt finger dissection we removed all the chest and abdominal organs. Scissors and scalpels were used to obtain small tissue specimens for later microscopic examination. An hour passed quickly. With a procedure to perform and instructions to follow my queasiness disappeared. I didn't realize it at the time, but the course of my life had changed.

A year later I had chosen a career path. I'd always done well in math and science and enjoyed solving difficult problems. There were three pathologists at Bronson Hospital I'd been assisting. They were well respected, enjoyed their work, and eager to start

11

every morning. They loved to teach, and enthusiastically shared their laboratory and autopsy results. Using scientific knowledge, performing procedures, making a diagnosis, medical decision making, I could see that medicine would be a challenging and rewarding career.

I grew up in the small town of Chelsea, Michigan. In the summer of 1970, our family moved. I attended Grosse Pointe South high school Junior and Senior years. Their calculus, chemistry and physics classes were tremendous. Freshman year at Kalamazoo College my grades were top notch, much of that year was a review. Sophomore year I slumped a bit. In addition to schoolwork, I participated in two varsity sports: diving and tennis. I enjoyed social activities, mostly chasing girls and partying on Friday and Saturday nights. My academic record showed the effects.

In my Junior year I worked at Bronson hospital, then went to Europe on the foreign study program. I decided on medicine as a career. First of course, I'd have to get accepted into medical school. I needed to improve my grades. Kalamazoo College was a small liberal arts college, academically competitive. I became a completely serious student, never missing class and waking up early. The campus breakfast hall and library were quiet lonely places before 10 AM, making it easy to concentrate and study. Out went most social activity, I went to bed before midnight. I lost a few friends, some complained that I was selfish. They were probably right, but there was no other way. I was pretty sharp but to get excellent grades I had to give 100 percent. I knew if I went partying and staying out late, then all the studying and facts I'd learned that day would be forgotten. I needed a good night's sleep to incorporate information into long term memory.

One dramatic turning point was in my second physical chemistry class. There were only 12 students, mostly physics and chemistry majors. The material and concepts were complex and difficult, but with extremely hard work I thought I was mastering it. There were only two exams, a midterm and final. The midterm was on a Friday. There were 12 questions, 25 points each, so the top score would be 300. We could take three hours. I thought I was prepared. The first three questions on page one were challenging, and I slowly worked them out. I turned to page two. Question four was: "Here is a blank periodic table. Fill it in." All the symbols, atomic numbers, and weights. Unbelievable! There were over one hundred different elements. We'd been working with the periodic table all semester, but no one had warned us about memorizing the whole thing. I surprised myself by coming up with about 40 of them, but knew I was in trouble. The rest of the midterm was similarly difficult. I was sweating. After three hours I was physically washed out and mentally exhausted. It was the most difficult exam I'd ever taken, by far.

Tuesday was the next class day and I waited anxiously. Tuesday morning came. When the professor walked in there was complete silence. Sounded and felt like dread. He handed each student their scored exam. I saw my total inscribed at the top of the first page: 129 (out of 300). What a disaster. I had trouble breathing. I must have been kidding myself, to think I could achieve enough academic success to consider medical school. I tried to fathom alternate careers. Maybe a science teacher, a taxi driver or tennis instructor. I struggled to think of other possibilities.

The professor walked to the chalk board and started writing the scores (without names). 142, 129, 107, 94, 91, 88, ….. down to 72. He explained that he'd given all A's and B's. He taught this course many times and knew ours was a class of talented students. He was tired of giving tests with everyone scoring above 90 percent. His goal was to challenge us, to see what we really knew. Totally relieved, I could breathe again. Within minutes I realized my determination and dedication was paying off. The possibility of a career in medicine was still viable. This wouldn't be the last time my emotions would swiftly change between despair and elation.

I mailed applications to six medical schools, getting accepted was difficult and extremely competitive. In a few weeks I received three rejections, but also three requests for interviews: University of Chicago, University of Michigan, and Wayne State University. The first two went well, and I was told the admission committees decisions would take four to six weeks. My third interview was a disaster. Arriving at Wayne State University I was told there had been a mix up. There was no one available to interview me. An hour later a hurried, slightly disheveled professor arrived. He briefly reviewed my application and curtly zipped through a few standard questions. He hardly looked up; I could tell he wasn't paying attention to my responses. After five minutes he glanced up and asked if I would like a tour. They might be able to find a medical student to show me around.

"Uh, no, that's alright," I replied. There was a limp handshake, the interview was over.

Weeks passed. Another rejection, from Chicago. Only two schools left. My mood matched the dark, cloudy, damp, dreary, late winter weather. On a Thursday afternoon things changed. There was a thick envelope in the mail from the University of Michigan. I had to read the first sentence twice. I was accepted into their medical school for the fall semester. Fantastic! My suitemates were whooping and hollering. I was near tears and could hardly speak.

––––––––––––––––

A week later I went home for an Easter visit. My folks were happy to see me. Thrilled with my acceptance to medical school they congratulated me over and over. They were so joyous I felt they almost couldn't believe it was true. Not because they thought I didn't have the talent or determination, but perhaps due to that small town doubt (that many of us had but would seldom admit) about making it in the big city. They had grown up in Newberry, Michigan in the 1930's, a town of about 2,500 people. I wondered if parents feel the joys of happy events (and the sadness of tragic ones) involving their children more intensely than their children themselves.

Hold On Tight

It was anatomy class, and I was struggling. Medical school curricula included two years of classes followed by two years of clinical rotations. The actual scientific concepts were not extremely difficult, but the amount of information was extraordinarily massive. Anatomy involved cadaver dissection and detailed study of the visible human structures. With my previous autopsy experience, I was adept at dissection. There was an enormous number of structures and relationships to learn. Take the forearm: 25 muscles in the forearm, each is located in a certain compartment, has an origin and insertion, an arterial blood supply and venous return, and unique innervation. That's 150 facts. We were supposed to learn all of this. I was overwhelmed with the task of memorization. My enthusiasm for classroom work rapidly diminished. I was passing but my low test scores accurately reflected my performance.

Dr. Vic Satori was a fifth-year senior surgical resident. He was our supervisor in the dissection lab. He was a busy, talented, no-nonsense physician. One Thursday I finally decided to ask for some direction. "Dr. Satori, I need help. I'm drowning with all the information in the anatomy manual. Look at this one page. There are about 40 names and structures. I can't possibly memorize it all."

He paused for a moment and said, "Let me tell you something. Big people think big. Little people think little." He went to the next dissection table.

What did that mean? "Big people think big." Sometimes seemingly minor details were important. How could I know what the important parts in anatomy were?

That evening I opened the anatomy instruction manual. About halfway down the page I noticed one structure was written in CAPITAL letters. On the entire page, out of 40 notations only four were capitalized. Every page was similar, only ten percent capitalized. Oh, my goodness. In my effort to be completely thorough and diligent I tried to master every single item. That was the wrong approach. I needed to concentrate on the big, important things. The next exam was scheduled for Monday. I spent most of my time learning the capitalized items. When the test started, I recognized about 90 percent of the questions involved the capitalized material. My struggles disappeared. It still wasn't easy, but my scores improved dramatically.

It was July of 1978. After two grueling years of classroom work, I began clinical rotations. My first month would be in the OB (Obstetrical) unit at Henry Ford Hospital. My parents lived nearby, so I spent the night before at their home. My mother was especially excited about me delivering a baby. She had ten children, nine cesarean sections (one set of twins). I awoke early, before the alarm went off. It was just getting light outside. I quickly dressed, grabbed my white medical student jacket, and quietly left the house. As I was getting into my car the back door of the house creaked open.

My mother called, "Mark, I need to tell you about the dream I had last night." Curious, I couldn't recall her ever telling us about a dream, I walked over to her. "I dreamt you were delivering your first baby, and you dropped it." There was a pause. I didn't know what to say. "I thought I'd better tell you."

"Oh. Well, thanks," I murmured, "I'll try and be careful." With that maternal vote of confidence, off I went. I prayed she wasn't clairvoyant.

I recall a few things about that OB rotation. I'd read and heard about the severe pain of contractions during labor but was unprepared for being at the bedside. Observing the tremendous discomfort at close range was dramatic. The absolute worst was spending a week with an obstetrician who specialized in the deliveries of young pregnant teenage women. Their long howling screams (a mixture of anxiety, fear, and severe pain) were at ear damaging decibels. These repeated every few minutes, intensifying as delivery approached. I concluded that OB was not my calling.

Twenty years later I was visiting my parents and recalled my mother's dream. "Mom, do you remember when I was in medical school, and you had a dream about me dropping a baby?"

"Oh, yes," she replied.

"Well, I've delivered about 50 babies (a few in medical school, many during Family Practice residency and a few in the ER). I wanted to let you know, I haven't dropped one yet!" I paused, quite proud of myself; waiting to hear some note of congratulations or maybe even a compliment about my technical skills.

She thought for a moment and said, "Well, maybe that's why," instantly deflating my boasting. She was probably right. I recalled paying special attention during obstetrical training about how to grasp a newborn infant (one hand behind the baby's neck and the other hand encircling one or both legs just above the ankles). She deserved most of the credit.

Residency Training

July 1st, 1980. My shift started at 6 PM in the ER. I was ready. After four long years of medical school, I was happy to be "Dr. Thomson," and eager to start. The head nurse gave me a brief tour, pointed out the chart rack of patients to be seen, then introduced me to Dr. Cook, a fifth-year surgery resident. He was running the ER that evening and would be my supervisor.

I grabbed the first chart. The chief complaint: "Shoulder Pain." I walked to room 23 and introduced myself, "Hi, I'm Dr. Thomson. Tell me about your shoulder." In front of me, sitting on the edge of the bed was a young woman who was obviously intoxicated. She was in a hospital gown. She was holding her right wrist with her left hand, to avoid any motion of her right arm. She smelled of alcohol, her conjunctival blood vessels were dilated, and her speech slurred. She had been walking away from an outdoor party and encountered a fence. She tried to climb over, fell, and hurt her right shoulder. She denied other injuries or pain.

I quickly examined her from head to toe. Nothing abnormal except for the alcohol. Examining the right arm, I didn't see any swelling, deformity, or bruising. Gently palpating her shoulder caused mild diffuse discomfort. Any range of motion however caused immediate severe pain with loud, long hollering. "We'll get a quick X-ray," I explained.

The shoulder X-rays returned, and I put the films up on a lighted view box. I inspected the films carefully and could not find any abnormality. Standing by the view box I presented the case. Dr. Cook listened impatiently to my history and physical exam. I thought the X-rays were normal and had no diagnosis except a possible sprained right shoulder. "Here's an obvious anterior shoulder dislocation," he pronounced, pointing to an area on the AP (frontal) X-ray view. I couldn't see it. "Look here on the lateral view," he said, motioning to the displaced proximal humerus (arm bone). I still couldn't see the dislocation. Wow. My beginner's confidence was evaporating rapidly.

Off we went to reduce the dislocated shoulder. Dr. Cook introduced himself to the young lady. He pointed to an area on her lateral right shoulder "See the swelling from the dislocated humeral head?"

"Uh, yes," I responded softly, not really sure.

"You get the first try," he said.

I'd seen one shoulder reduction as a medical student. This would be my first attempt. The nurse gave 50 mg of Demerol IV (intravenous) push. After a minute I applied gentle inline traction, holding her wrist and pulling on her right arm. The young woman screamed in agony. Nothing happened to the dislocation.

"Pull harder," was Dr. Cook's instruction.

I did. There was another painful scream. Again, nothing happened by the right shoulder.

Dr. Cook rolled his eyes in disgust, "Enough, I'll do it."

I lowered my head and stepped away, my self-esteem in tatters. He placed his right heel into the patient's right axilla (armpit), grabbed her right wrist and gave a tremendous yank. She screamed louder and more intensely. Nothing happened by her right shoulder. Dr.

Cook pulled again, rotating the arm back and forth for almost a minute. I didn't think it was humanly possible to scream so loud.

After he finally stopped the second attempt the young woman finished her anguished holler and yelled out, "My elbow!!!"

I carefully inspected her right elbow. There was a small but obvious swelling posteriorly. Gently palpating I could easily feel the dislocated olecranon (back point of the elbow). Oh my goodness. The shoulder had never been dislocated; she had a dislocated elbow in the first place. She must have referred pain to the shoulder. A well-known phenomenon (to experienced physicians). I had completely missed the diagnosis, focusing too much on the complaint of shoulder pain. I hadn't carefully examined the elbow. A common, rookie mistake.

Dr. Cook disappeared. I ordered X-rays of the elbow; they confirmed the elbow dislocation. There was no fracture. I was able to reduce the dislocated elbow on the first attempt. There was moderate (but significantly less) screaming. Under the watchful eyes of an experienced ER tech, I placed a posterior plaster splint. She made me remove it. Then graciously took the time to teach me how to properly add padding to protect the injured joint. Post reduction X-rays were normal, the elbow joint was in good position.

I prepared the discharge instructions. Her friends arrived to take her home. The patient was less intoxicated by this time. She didn't seem to remember me pulling on her arm. She was quite thankful about me reducing the elbow dislocation. I learned so many lessons from my first patient it was hard to think of them all. Don't anchor so much on the initial complaint. Do a careful, thorough physical exam. Consider other injuries if the history, physical exam, and X-rays don't match. Speak up if there's disagreement on interpreting the imaging studies. It is difficult to know what you don't know. Have a healthy skepticism for pronouncements from hot shot senior resident physicians.

My next rotation was in the ICU (Intensive Care Unit). I learned how to insert a central IV line. Most patients in the ICU required blood draws, numerous IV medications and fluids. This could easily be accomplished through one large IV in a central vein. Common sites for these catheters were femoral (near the groin) or subclavian (under the clavicle) veins. The femoral site was good but had a high rate of infection. The subclavian route became the preferred site. The "Seldinger Technique" was straightforward. The physician would use sterile gloves, prep a wide area near the clavicle with betadine and place sterile drapes. You would palpate the clavicle, insert a long 14-gauge (large diameter) needle attached to a syringe, under the clavicle and aim for the sternal notch. You pull the barrel of the syringe back a bit and slowly advance the needle. After a few centimeters there would be a sudden gush of dark blood, confirming entrance to the subclavian vein. The syringe would be removed, a thin guidewire advanced through the needle, and then the needle withdrawn. A small nick incision of the skin was made with a scalpel, a large catheter threaded over the wire into position in the subclavian vein, then the wire was then removed. The catheter sewn into place and IV attached.

There are three fairly common complications. One: inadvertent poking of the subclavian artery. The artery is adjacent to the vein, and if punctured is easy to recognize. Arterial blood is bright red, pulsates and spurts out the needle tip when you remove the syringe to insert the wire. This can be avoided by keeping the tip of the needle exactly next to the clavicle during insertion as the vein is located close to the clavicular bone. If patients were on blood thinning medication you choose the femoral vein route. The artery is near a vein as well, but pressure to stop arterial bleeding is easily applied. Two: infection. This is a late complication. The rate of infection can be decreased by paying strict attention to sterile techniques. Three: a collapsed lung or pneumothorax. The lung is close to the clavicle, but by palpating the clavicle and keeping the needle next to its posterior edge the incidence of damaging the lung is small.

We documented our procedures. I was feeling good about my subclavian access. I'd done 20 of them without complication. One day at morning rounds another resident asked if I could place a central line on an 87-year-old patient of his. The patient was scheduled for major surgery later that day. "Not a problem, happy to," I replied. I loved performing procedures.

A short time later I was in the middle of the procedure. I advanced the 14-gauge needle under the right clavicle. I suddenly aspirated about 2 cc's of air, followed by dark red blood. I'd certainly nicked the lung. I knew that was easy to do, especially on thin elderly patients where there wasn't much tissue between the subclavian vein and the top of the lung. I quickly passed the wire and placed the large bore IV catheter. I confirmed a good catheter position by aspirating blood from all three ports. I ordered the routine portable chest X-ray as a STAT (immediate) study, concerned about a possible pneumothorax.

I stayed at the bedside. Within two minutes the patient developed severe respiratory distress with rapid breathing, and tachycardia (a fast heart rate). I listened to his lungs. There were no breath sounds on the right. He had a large pneumothorax. I checked the neck and found swollen jugular veins indicating increase pressure in his chest. This was a life-threatening tension pneumothorax! I ran and grabbed a chest tube tray and asked for a nurse to join me. I'd only placed one chest tube before, and this man needed one immediately. He could crash and die at any moment. I opened the tray and glanced up hearing the portable X-ray machine coming into the patient's room. Just beyond the machine I saw Dr. Ferguson walking past. Dr. Ferguson was a talented physician (the chief resident in general surgery). He'd always been pleasant to work with, coming quickly to the ICU when we needed consultation or a procedure. He was calm and collected, no matter how critical the situation.

"Dr. Ferguson, can you help me?" I hollered out to him.

He stepped into the room, "What's the problem Mark?" he asked calmly. He examined the patient. I told him I had just placed a subclavian catheter and thought I caused a tension pneumothorax.

He paused for a few seconds, then reached over and grabbed the scalpel with his right hand. With his left hand he palpated the patient's right axilla, then plunged the scalpel through the chest wall. Immediately a large gush of air rushed out of the chest. In seconds the respiratory distress disappeared. The rapid breathing and heart rate resolved. He had saved the patient's life. Dr. Ferguson had been in the room for about 90 seconds. He took a few minutes and skillfully inserted a chest tube. The chest X-ray confirmed excellent placement and a beautifully expanded right lung.

What a fantastic stroke of luck that Dr. Ferguson had been walking by. I might have been able to relieve the patient's tension pneumothorax, but it would have been close. I looked back at the patient; he was frail and weak. He had dementia. I don't think he even knew what occurred. I knew. I'd put a patient in grave danger. I gained a new perspective on a, "Low Rate" of complications. After 20 central lines without a problem, I'd become far too cavalier. If a patient was having the complication the rate was 100 percent for them. I resolved a couple things: I wouldn't start a procedure until I was certain I was comfortable handling complications, and I would call for help and consultations early. Long before my patient was near death.

Early in my career I was extremely confident. After years of education, I felt well trained, had good procedural skills, and could handle any challenge in caring for patients. While moonlighting in the Novi ER Mrs. Williams, an 82-year-old woman, arrived with significant shortness of breath (SOB). The triage nurse placed her into room 1, which also served as our resuscitation room. Mrs.

Williams had a history of heart disease and congestive heart failure (CHF). This occurs when the heart muscle is damaged and weak, then can no longer pump blood effectively. Fluid backs up into the lungs causing SOB. Normally, the lungs are soft and pliable. They expand and contract with each breath, easily moving air in and out. This allows oxygen to dissolve into the blood, and carbon dioxide to be removed and exhaled. This process can be markedly impaired if the lungs get congested from fluid or infection. The lungs get stiff and the work of breathing increases. A large amount of fluid can lead to respiratory failure. Patients may require intubation (a breathing tube inserted into the trachea). A ventilator (breathing machine) forces air into the lungs under pressure, significantly improving lung function.

This was a common problem; I'd seen CHF cases frequently. Mrs. Williams' past medical history was remarkable for hypertension and rheumatoid arthritis. Her surgical history included a hip replacement 6 months before after a fall and hip fracture. She was on 16 medications including a beta blocker (a drug that slows the heart rate). On exam she was a frail elderly woman, mildly pale and struggling to breath. Upon auscultation of her posterior chest, I found fluid about a third of the way up from the diaphragm to the top of her shoulders. Fluids tend to settle from gravity. In CHF it accumulates first just above the diaphragm then rises. Mrs. Williams pulse oxygen measurement was 89 % when she arrived (normal is 96-100 %).

We placed her on oxygen via nasal cannula (NC). The pulse ox improved to 94 %. I ordered a diuretic, (to help the kidneys excrete fluid) and since her blood pressure was high a couple inches of nitro paste. A foley catheter was inserted into the bladder to monitor and collect urine output. A portable chest X-ray confirmed the fluid congestion in the chest. On repeat examination she had improved, her pulse ox measured 96 %, respiratory rate 26 (normal 12 to 20), and heart rate 102 (normal 60 to 100). She needed to be admitted for further management. I paged her internist and planned a transfer to the inpatient hospital. EMS (an ambulance with trained paramedics) was called. They would arrive in about 20 minutes. The transfer driving time to the inpatient hospital was 30 minutes.

I was charting into the Med Rec (medical record) when Peggy, her RN (registered nurse), stopped by.

"Aren't you going to intubate the patient in Room 1?" she asked.

"Mrs. Williams?" I asked, a bit surprised. I thought the patient was stable and so hadn't planned on intubation.

"She doesn't look good to me. I think she's going to tire out," Peggy said.

This concerned me. Peggy had tons of experience, having worked in the ER for many years. "I'll circle back and check on her." I rechecked the patient and couldn't see any worsening. I told Peggy, "She looks okay to me. I'll check again when EMS gets here."

About 30 minutes later EMS arrived. Peggy called me into room 1. The paramedics were starting to take patient report (pertinent clinical details) from Peggy. Mrs. Williams however was looking worse. She was a little confused, had mild cyanosis (bluish discoloration) of her lips, was sitting forward in the bed, using accessory muscles in her chest and neck to help with breathing. Her oxygen reading had dropped to 90 %, RR (Respiratory rate)

30, and HR (Heart rate) 116. Not horrible, but Peggy was right. Chest auscultation showed the fluid now halfway up the chest. The elderly woman was about to "Crash" (suddenly decompensate and become critically ill).

"Let's get her intubated," I said. I ordered succinylcholine (a short acting paralytic medication). Without deep sedation or paralysis, the vocal cords close during intubation, due to stimulation and reflexes in the back of the throat. I placed the endotracheal tube without difficulty and connected it to a ventilator. We suctioned a large amount of frothy pink fluid from the trachea. I ordered 5 cm of PEEP (positive end-expiratory pressure with ventilation). In the few minutes it took to obtain a portable chest X-ray, Mrs. Williams was looking much better. Oxygen was 98 %, heart rate of 100, and a good flow of urine was draining into the collection bag.

This could have been a disaster. It was fortunate the EMS unit was slow to arrive. If this patient had "Crashed" in the EMS unit, it would have been quite dangerous. There is only one paramedic with the patient (the other driving). Intubation by one person in a moving vehicle can be exceedingly difficult. In the ER we typically have three team members: an RN giving medications, the Respiratory Therapist (RT) assisting and managing ventilation, and the physician performing intubation.

Peggy had been clairvoyant. "How did you know this patient might crash?" I asked. "She didn't look that bad to me."

"Well," Peggy said slowly, "She was so thin and frail, and wasn't making any urine."

I was getting an education. I recalled the history of hip fracture. Many elderly patients fall and break their hips from general debility and have a life expectancy of less than one year. Mrs. Williams didn't have extra lung or heart capacity. Her good oxygen level was only because we placed her on high flow oxygen. Also, it hadn't occurred to me that the beta blocker prevented a faster heart rate (which may have indicated an unstable patient). "Peggy, you might have just saved her life. Thank you." I had better wake up. I had much to learn.

During my third and last year of family practice residency I was rotating through a Pediatric office practice, supervised by Dr. Gleason and three other experienced pediatricians. They were talented and enthusiastic teachers. The month-long rotation had come highly recommended. One fall afternoon a mother raced in with her 10-year-old daughter. The child had crashed while riding her bike, flying forward over the handlebars. There were obvious head and facial injuries, an actively bleeding forehead laceration, and a swollen and painful right shoulder. Acute pediatric trauma patients with anything more than a minor injury were quite unusual in the office setting. Dr. Gleason was about to call for an EMS unit for transfer when he remembered me calling him from the ER regarding one of his patients needing hospital admission.

"How long have you been moonlighting in the ER," he asked?

"One night a week for about a year," I said. He wondered if I would take a quick look at the child. "Of course."

I checked the child's VS (vital signs: temperature, respiratory rate, heart rate and blood pressure) while getting a brief history. The initial trauma survey indicated no serious or critical injuries. The secondary head to toe exam revealed a contusion to the head, the deep forehead laceration (bleeding controlled easily with direct pressure), facial abrasions and bruising without crepitus or deformity (ruling out facial bone fracture) and swelling, tenderness, and deformity over the mid right clavicle (indicating a fracture). I placed her right arm in a sling for comfort and asked if they had a suture kit available.

Then I noticed the Pediatricians watching me from the hall. They hadn't seen much trauma since finishing their residency training five to ten years previously. I explained my evaluation to the young patient and her mother. My straightforward approach had a calming effect. In the ER I had seen many similar cases. The laceration repair went smoothly. It was deep, right to the bone (common in this area), but there was no foreign material. After slowly injecting local anesthesia (to minimize discomfort), I irrigated the wound, reapproximated the wound margins with sutures, applied antibiotic ointment and a gauze dressing. The clavicular fracture was confirmed by X-ray. I gave routine instructions, and the mother and child were on their way.

It was an enjoyable experience. The mother and Pediatricians were thankful. I was using my recently obtained knowledge and technical skills. Emergency patients typically need a brief but focused history, a careful and detailed physical examination, often followed by a few chosen laboratory tests and / or imaging studies.

A diagnosis is made, and treatment started. Procedures are common (splinting and laceration repair in this case) and provide immediate benefit and pain relief. Nearly all emergency patients were thankful. I found this type of medical practice interesting and satisfying.

Months later I went to a few small towns in northern Michigan, looking for a place to start a Family Practice. My wife accompanied me. We met during my sophomore year of medical school and married two years later. We quickly grew our family (adding three children in four years). She was aghast at the lack of activities available near these remote locations. She had been raised in the suburban Detroit area. My childhood was in Chelsea, Michigan, population about 3,000. I knew that being a physician in a small town would be rewarding, you would be a respected and integral part of the community. She knew I loved hiking and fishing. She worried (correctly) that I might leave her alone at home, far from her close-knit family, with our small children.

About that time the owner of the EM (Emergency Medicine) physician group, where I was moonlighting, offered me a contract. I considered a career change. I enjoyed practicing medicine in the ER, the specialty of EM was developing. I could become board certified in emergency medicine after five years without having to complete another residency. We could live nearby in a rural area, but close to big city amenities. The decision was easy. I signed the contract. I would be an EM physician.

Meningitis

Dr. Simpson was giving the morning sign-out report, telling me about a patient in the ER from his midnight shift. In the early 1980's our ER was typically slow after 1 AM. It had been a quiet night; the only patient left was a 6-month-old female infant. She was brought in by her mother, arriving 30 minutes before. The chief complaint was fever and crying.

Dr. Simpson said, "I couldn't find anything on the exam. She's quiet now, sucking on a pacifier. I ordered some lab tests, a urine analysis (UA), and a chest X-ray. Would you check on the results for me?"

"Of course. No problem. Drive home safely."

Marsha, the midnight RN, stopped by my desk immediately after sign-out. "Would you check this baby? She doesn't look right," she asked urgently. Marsha was a skilled and experienced RN. She could recognize a patient who only had subtle signs of serious illness. I trusted her intuition. I went straight to the baby's room. The mother was standing nervously next to the crib. They had just returned from radiology. The mother told me she was a healthy baby, her only child. This was the infant's first illness. Yesterday evening she felt warm, became fussy and would only breastfeed a short time. The last two hours she wouldn't stop crying.

While listening to the history, I'd been observing the child. What I saw scared me. The infant was lying on its back, occasionally sucking on a pacifier. She was not in marked distress and appeared to be sleeping. Her breathing was fast, about 48 times a minute. With each expiration I could hear a soft grunt. This was a subtle but significant sign of respiratory distress. Looking closely at the top of her head there was mild swelling of the anterior fontanelle (soft spot). I bumped the crib gently while lowering the rail to examine the child. That shook the baby, and immediately she started to cry. A high pitched, distressing cry. With fever, irritability, and the bulging fontanelle the only likely diagnosis was meningitis. This infant was critically ill.

We were able to do the septic work up quickly. Marsha started the IV and drew blood cultures while I opened the LP (lumbar puncture) kit for a spinal tap. During the LP the infant was restrained on its side. I noticed mild cyanosis of the hands and feet, this resolved quickly. Of grave concern, the spinal fluid was cloudy indicating meningitis. We dispensed with the urine catheterization. Marsha gave IV Ceftriaxone (an antibiotic). I walked the spinal fluid samples to the lab.

"Can you do a Gram stain right away?" I asked.

"Certainly," Teri, our lab technician said, "I'll call you as soon as it's done." I went back to the ER and made a few calls to arrange admission.

Teri called back, "Dr. Thomson, you'd better come take a look at the slide." Taking turns at the microscope, we examined the spinal fluid. I didn't want to believe it. The whole field of view was filled with thousands of lancet-shaped (elongated round) cocci in pairs. The walls of the bacteria were dark from the Gram stain. There were only a few WBC's (White Blood Cells) present, a weak immune response.

"Pneumococcus?" I asked Teri.

34

"It has to be," she replied.

The EMS unit arrived. I went into the room and talked with the mother, "This is meningitis, a serious infection around the brain." The mother was terrified, quiet, and tearful. So were the day shift nurses who'd arrived. "It's very dangerous, but we've given a powerful antibiotic. We can hope for a good response," I explained. I tried to sound optimistic. The infant was transferred to the Pediatric ICU.

"What happened? How could the baby get critically ill so quickly?" asked the nurses.

"I've read about Pneumococcus. It's a common bacterium that we are all exposed to, even carry in the back of our throat. It typically causes ear and throat infections, and occasionally pneumonia. But it can do strange things, there are many different strains. For some reason in some patients, it can cause rapid overwhelming infections. This infant needs a miracle," I explained, trying to prepare them for a likely bad outcome. Two days later we received a call back from the Pediatric ICU. The infant had quickly developed septic shock. Cultures of blood and spinal fluid grew Pneumococcus. The antibiotic had no effect. The baby died 12 hours after arrival to their unit.

You're The Doctor?

Julie was a young woman sitting on our fast-track bench near the X-ray view box, a spot reserved for healthy patients with minor injuries. These patients were seen by our ER triage nurse who ordered plain X-rays. The patient would go directly to the radiology department, and then return to the ER and be asked to sit on the bench. Their X-ray films would be placed in a folder and tucked in a slot just underneath the view box. I grabbed her chart from the rack and reviewed it briefly. Fall, injured right wrist was the chief complaint.

"Are you Julie? I'm Dr. Thomson."

She paused, then replied slowly, "Yes, yes. I am." She eyed me suspiciously.

"Tell me how you hurt your wrist."

"You, you're the Doctor? Here in the emergency room?" She seemed shocked.

"Yes, of course," I replied calmly. Julie looked like she didn't believe me.

I'd been working in the ER for a few years. I was fortunate to look young for my age. A few patients (typically older) seemed hesitant about allowing me to care for them. So, I had changed from wearing the green hospital scrubs to a shirt and tie under my white lab coat. Later, I returned to scrubs (too much blood and contamination), but by then some gray hair helped convince patients that their ER doctor might have enough experience.

Julie remained hesitant, a small, concerned frown persisted.

"Tell me what happened," I encouraged her.

"Well, ookaayy," Julie began. "I got out of my car, took a few steps, and slipped on some ice. I fell on my right wrist." She denied any other pain or injuries. I explained how we see many similar injuries after an ice storm turns to snow. The hidden ice causes numerous falls.

I knelt in front of her to examine the injured area. She cautiously extended her right wrist forward. The skin was intact, gentle ROM (range of motion) of the shoulder, elbow, wrist, and hand was painless. There was localized tenderness to gentle palpation on both the dorsal and volar aspects (top and bottom) of her distal radius (a bone just proximal to the wrist). There was no tenderness over the navicular bone or with thumb compression (ruling out an easy to miss navicular fracture).

"Let's have a look at your X-rays," I said. The films had already been placed up on the illuminated view box. There was a small slightly irregular line in the distal radius, an undisplaced fracture. The fracture line didn't enter the joint space. This was fortunate, as fractures into the joint can heal slowly and occasionally lead to arthritic complications. Her fracture would heal beautifully in four to six weeks.

I turned back to Julie and started to explain the fracture and the plaster splint we would apply. She seemed completely baffled by this information and suddenly blurted out, "Wait, wait! Do YOU have a BROTHER who TEACHES at Wayne State University?"

Now I was surprised. "Oh. Yes. I do. Michael Thomson is my brother."

Julie let out a long sigh in relief and said, "When I was signing in, I heard and recognized your voice. At first, I couldn't place it, but then I realized it sounded exactly like my economics professor Dr. Thomson. I didn't think he could be an ER doctor, but I looked at my wrist band and it said, "Dr. Thomson." So, I guess it was possible. He is a "Doctor." I was sitting here, you walked by, and you look like him. I could hardly believe that my economics professor was also a medical doctor. So, I had to ask."

"No problem," I assured her. "We're identical twins. Most of our friends can hardly tell us apart, especially our voices. Even I have difficulty when I see us in a home movie." Julie was much happier, now that her economics professor wasn't treating her in the ER. I placed a plaster splint, gave routine instructions, and merrily sent her on her way.

———————————

About 2 AM a group of young adults brought in their friend Doug for evaluation. They had been to a bar and drinking a fair amount of alcohol. At some point Doug had told them he was considering killing himself. I was able to obtain some history from the friends, and a bit from the obviously intoxicated patient himself. He was single, struggling at work, had no prior history of depression, mental illness, or suicide attempts. He had no medical problems (except for binge drinking on weekends.)

On examination, Doug had markedly slurred speech and couldn't answer many questions.

He would have to be held in the ER to "Sober up." He was placed in room 10 (close to the nurses' station) and put in a hospital gown. His clothes and possessions were taken out of the room, and he had one wrist and ankle strapped to the bed frame. He wasn't happy with the restraints but didn't struggle. I briefly explained to Doug that we had to follow ER protocol. After a short while he fell asleep. The staff checked on him frequently.

A challenge for physicians is assessment of suicide potential in ER patients. It was well described in the medical literature that many significantly depressed and / or mentally ill patients who go on to commit suicide visit their family doctor or an ER in the days or weeks before taking their life. It was hoped health care providers could identify patients at risk and start treatment or interventions to prevent tragic outcomes.

Trying to predict future behavior of anyone is difficult, and among widely variable patient presentations to the ER it can be nearly impossible. I could group patients into three categories. Obviously suicidal: someone addicted to alcohol or drugs who had recently been thrown out of the house, lost their job, purchased a firearm, and wrote a note about their plan and goal to end it all. Obviously not suicidal: a young adult with no history of addiction or mental illness, had good friends and family support, no history of prior attempts, no concrete plan, and briefly stated they didn't want to live after a fight with their boyfriend or girlfriend. The majority of my potentially suicidal ER patients fell between those two extremes, and their suicide risk was difficult to estimate. Any intoxicating effects of alcohol or drugs need to be minimal to accurately assess patients.

Over time, the ER had a widely variable restraint policy for suicidal patients. It was restrain everyone, alternating with do not restrain anyone. Of course, the humane thing is to never restrain anyone. Which policy we followed was dictated by the hospitals' legal advisors and recent occurrences. When I began practicing, we restrained all patients who had more than minimal risk of suicide. This was because of numerous lawsuits (in the early 1980's) involving patients running out of a hospital ER, heading to the nearest roadway, and jumping off a bridge or into highway traffic and committing suicide.

After 6 to 12 months of restraining our ER patients enough complaints and threats of lawsuits would filter up through the hospital administration that the policy was changed back to restraining almost no one. We had been asked (more than once) to only restrain those patients about to "Elope" from the ER. We pointed out that none of us could predict which patients were about to elope.

One memorable occurrence involved a young unrestrained woman. She was low risk and had been placed in a hospital gown and her belongings taken from the room. It was 7:30 AM, we were awaiting the social worker to arrive. Unexpectedly she bolted from the room and out the ambulance entrance. One of our middle-aged nurses took off running in pursuit. I was called over to the door with other staff members and watched as the patient headed towards the nearest roadway. The patient's gown was billowing open, we could see her naked back side. The young woman was a fast runner and easily left the RN behind. We lost sight of them heading over a berm. Soon, the short of breath nurse returned.

"What happened?" we asked.

"You wouldn't believe it. When she got to the road there was a bunch of traffic. The first car she waved down stopped and picked her up! Off they went." Briefly, I wondered who would stop for a nearly naked, running young woman, dressed only in a hospital gown? Later that afternoon the patient responded to our telephone calls. She returned to the ER for her clothes and had a discussion with our social worker. Plans were made for close outpatient follow up.

Nowadays the ER restraint issue is addressed with a somewhat costly solution. A human "Sitter" is assigned to each at-risk patient and stays either at the bedside or just outside the patient's room. A security guard is posted by the ER entrances as well. Restraints are rarely used.

Back to Doug. About 6 AM a bemused nurse came to my desk. "You know the patient in room 10?"

"Of course," I replied.

Well, he just told me, "Go get that little asshole Mexican doctor. Tell him I want to talk to him." She started laughing hysterically.

How about that? Even though the patient appeared markedly intoxicated when he arrived, his assessment of me wasn't far off. I'm 5 ft 8 inches tall, and I was abrupt with him (the ER was busy, and my instructions to inebriated individuals were usually brief).

However, I'm not Mexican. I'm Italian with some French and English, and proud of it.

I went to see him. "Take these restraints off," he demanded. He was now thinking more clearly. I was able to have a discussion with him, and determined he was at low risk of suicide. A friend would come and get him from the ER. He assured me that he would follow up closely with his PCP (Primary Care Physician). We removed the restraints.

The nurses wouldn't let me forget this incident. The lead topic at shift change report that day was the patient from room 10, and his request for Dr. Thomson. He was quoted exactly, many times. After a couple days I forgot about the episode but should have known better. As per our routine schedule, I had worked four night shifts in a row, followed by four days off. Arriving about 6:45 AM for the first of my four day shifts, I noticed the staff oddly watching me as I walked to my office. There, in the center of my desk, was a tiny Mexican sombrero.

Shaken

"Dr. Thomson, come quick," called Carol the triage nurse. The urgency in her voice was unmistakable. A young woman had brought a 15-month-old child to the front entrance. Carol raced them to Resuscitation Room 1. The infant was unresponsive, dressed in pajama bottoms. He was pale, cold, and breathing only six times a minute. The team sprang into action: simultaneously undressing him, starting two IV lines, placing heart rate and oxygen monitors, administering blow by oxygen, and bringing warm blankets.

I began my exam and asked the mother, "What happened?"

"I don't know," she said. "He was fine last night when we went to bed. We found him lying on the bedroom floor when we woke up."

Something didn't seem right, it was 11:20 AM. Parents with young children typically don't sleep past 10 AM. "Who all was in the house last night?" I asked.

"Just me, my husband and our two children."

The child's airway was clear, the breathing was slow and shallow, the heart rate 100, pulse ox 90 % on the blow by oxygen. He was hypothermic, the rectal temperature 94 degrees (normal is 98.6). There were multiple bruises of different colors on the head, chest, arms and legs, a few small circular scars on the chest and back (likely old cigarette burns). There was an unusual imprint on the back. A dozen parallel lines 4 to 5 cm long indented the skin over the left posterior chest. The pupils were fixed and dilated.

Fundoscopic exam showed diffuse splotchy red patches on both retina (bilateral hemorrhages). I finished my exam.

The father arrived (from parking the car).

"What did you see," I asked.

"Nothing. We found him on the floor," the father replied.

"Was he lying on the register vent?" I asked.

"I think so."

That could explain the unusual imprint on the back. The child must have been lethargic and not moving for hours, to cause indentations like that. "Something happened. You have to tell me what happened," I demanded.

"What are you accusing me of, nothing happened," the father replied angrily.

I tried again. "No. You don't wake up to find your child like this. He's in a coma, and likely has bleeding on the brain. I'm trying to save his life. I need to know what happened." The parents were silent, the father hostile and glaring. "You can sit on that bench in the hall," I pointed. I noticed another child with them, about 5-years-old. I turned to a tech, "Ask security to keep an eye on them. Let me know if they leave." This infant had three suspicious injuries without any good story to explain them. It had to be traumatic abuse.

I intubated the child without any sedative or paralytic medication, he was deeply comatose. We sent off the routine traumatic lab panel and called the Pediatric ICU for transfer and admission. It was going to be 30 minutes for the EMS unit to arrive. We obtained a CT (computerized tomography) of the head and a skeletal X-ray survey. The CT showed intracranial bleeding and significant cerebral edema (swelling). The X-rays showed four old, healing rib fractures. The child's VS improved and stabilized; the temperature rose to 98 degrees with warm blankets.

It didn't matter. He was likely brain dead. Who would beat or shake a 15-month-old child to death? The transfer team arrived and quickly looked the infant over. I walked down the hall and spoke with the parents. "His VS are stable, but he has serious bleeding around the brain. I'm not sure he will make it." They acted concerned.

The EMS unit left with the infant. I called to report the case to DHHS (Department of Health and Human Services) and filled out the 3200 forms (suspected abuse). The ER had backed up. Caring for numerous patients I stayed busy for the rest of my shift.

Arriving home that evening about 6 PM, my sister-in-law Loretta and her husband Gary were visiting with their four young children. Our own children were the same age. They were running around, playing, screaming, and laughing. I still had green scrubs on. Loretta asked, "How was your day?" We were over to one side of the room, on the edge of the joyous activity.

There were some ER stories I couldn't tell. Loretta was a nurse, maybe she would understand. "Not so good today," I started and took a couple of deep breaths. "I saw a one-year-old," I started to shake, "Someone beat him to death." I broke down, leaned against the wall, bowed my head, and cried quietly. There was no way I could understand.

Later, I learned that one of the parents admitted to shaking the child. After two days in the Pediatric ICU the infant was declared brain dead and disconnected from the ventilator. There was a court case. I received a subpoena to appear, but after a plea bargain, I wasn't called to testify. As a witnessing physician I had been on the stand a few times and didn't find it stressful. Testifying didn't compare to the immediate aftermath of events in the ER.

Prepared

The Paramedics called enroute with, "A 10-year-old girl who fell off the monkey bars at school. She has an open (visible bone) fracture of the right humerus (arm)." They found no other injuries, established an IV and brought her to our ER. Surprisingly, upon arrival, the young girl was sitting innocently and calmly on the cart. One EMT (Emergency Medical Technician) kept her looking to the left. We slid her onto our ER bed and placed her into a hospital gown. The VS were normal. Remarkably, she appeared pain free. The initial trauma exam was negative. Her head, neck, facial bones, spine, chest, abdomen, pelvis, and other extremities were nontender.

Her mother arrived and entered the room. The only injury was her right humerus. Removing the splint and large bulky gauze wrap (placed by the paramedics) revealed an unusual fracture. About 10 cm (4 inches) of the shaft of the distal portion of the humerus was protruding towards the shoulder, completely exposed, and covered in coarse gravel. There was minimal bleeding. The arm was shortened four inches. There was significant swelling and bruising just above the elbow joint.

I had seen a fair number of open fractures; this was the most bone exposed ever. A couple staff members became pale. She could wiggle her fingers. Most concerning was that the child's right hand was pale and cold. The radial pulse was weakly palpable, the blood flow diminished by doppler (a handheld ultrasound device). This was a true emergency. Decreased blood flow causes a lack of oxygen. Serious tissue death could happen quickly, and permanent disability result. The right brachial artery near the elbow was likely injured or compressed. The young girl's lack of pain was from the displaced bone ends not touching (which would have been severely painful), and anesthesia (lack of sensation) distally from the lack of perfusion (blood flow) and oxygenation.

"We'll have to reduce the fracture as soon as possible." I had the mother sit on a chair in the corner. Five mg of morphine was given IV push for pain control and sedation. We rinsed the entire exposed bone with four liters (one gallon) of saline and gently brushed with sterile gauze pads. Keeping the child's head turned away she didn't even wince, oblivious to what the team was doing. Not exactly sure of the technique, I had a tech hold the right shoulder for stability, then firmly pulled her wrist with in-line traction. The exposed bone slid partially back through the wound. With more traction the humeral end disappeared. Keeping firm traction, I checked the alignment. I pronated (rotated inward) the forearm a little, the alignment improved. We checked the right radial pulse; it was much stronger! We placed the arm in a long posterior plaster splint. Rechecking the pulse, it was normal (equal to the left side). The repeat X-ray showed the humerus fracture with good alignment.

The on-call orthopedic surgeon returned my call. The young girl was boarded for surgery for a thorough wash out. After she was transferred a tech came by and asked, "Did you ever see a fracture like that? How did you know what to do?"

"First one," I said. "I was taught that you could seldom go wrong with in-line traction. It worked!" What was the quote from Louis Pasteur? "Chance favors the prepared mind." We were prepared that day.

Oh great. That's a problem. I had just stuck my left hand with a spinal needle. The patient had AIDS (Autoimmune deficiency syndrome) which was 100 % fatal. Now I was at risk.

The year was 1989. AIDS was a blood born (carried in the blood) infection caused by HIV (human immunodeficiency virus). Similar to hepatitis it was transmitted through sexual activity and infected needles. Healthcare workers were not a great risk, except by exposure to a patient's blood. The larger the amount of blood one was exposed to the higher the risk of becoming infected. At that time, there was no prophylactic antiviral medication. Once infected, there was no treatment. Infected individuals died within a few months to a few years.

My patient presented with a high fever, headache, weakness, and a history of AIDS. He was quiet and reserved. AIDS patients were treated like lepers, socially avoided, and rejected. Even knowing that casual contact wouldn't transmit the HIV virus it was difficult for many people to interact with AIDS patients. A disease that is 100 % fatal and exclusively found in homosexual men or IV drug users will do that. I made an extra effort to be courteous and understanding, to demonstrate (to the ER staff) that routine interactions such as shaking hands, taking BP (blood pressure), or palpating the abdomen carried no risk. There was no need to gown and glove except when doing procedures or being exposed to body fluids.

 He was pale, thin, and seriously ill. He needed the full septic work up with blood, urine, and spinal fluid cultures. I followed the same precautions for his spinal tap that I had always done (over 100 times before). The only change was putting on two sets of gloves. The procedure went smoothly. I placed the spinal needle in the L3 - L4 (lumbar 3 - 4) interspace about three cm deep and easily entered the spinal canal. The spinal fluid appeared clear (microscopic exam would show an infection). Before removing the needle, I placed my left hand near the puncture site. I don't know why; I had never done that before. Somehow, I thought I was being extra careful. I pulled the needle out slowly with my right hand. Just as the needle cleared the skin, the patient gave a big jerk. I never had a patient do that before, removing the needle slowly was usually painless. It surprised me.

The needle tip hit my left thumb, and I felt a prick. I removed my gloves and looked. I couldn't see a puncture wound and there was not a spec of blood. There was no syringe on the spinal needle. But there was no question. I felt the needle prick. I had been exposed to a microscopic amount of spinal fluid and possibly blood. I was angry for a moment. Why had he jerked? That quickly passed. It was my fault (putting my left hand near the sharp needle). I washed my hands thoroughly, then scrubbed with alcohol and betadine for good measure.

I sent his spinal fluid to the laboratory for analysis, then had a chart made out for myself. We followed the blood born (needle stick) exposure guidelines. In this case it would be more for documentation than anything. It was difficult to concentrate the rest of the day. I felt I was a dedicated physician. I had to see every patient presenting to the ER. I understood my life was at risk. Now, I worried about my wife and four small children. All I could do was wait six months to see if I became infected. I was glad to have life insurance.

The patient had cryptococcal meningitis. We started IV fluids, antibiotics, and antifungal medications. He was transferred to the ICU. He died approximately 10 days later.

I can understand any healthcare worker that would hesitate to come to work if patients have severe easily transmissible infections. Especially if the hospital or office did not have enough PPE (personal protective equipment: gowns, gloves, masks, etc). Continuing to care for patients in that situation reveals true courage and dedication.

Over the next six months my tests remained negative. I was fortunate. I never became infected.

Oral Board Examination

Waiting to start the EM oral board examination I was nervous. Really, really, nervous. I was in the lobby on the sixth floor of a hotel near the Chicago airport. Milling about and pacing around with me were 20 other physicians. After four years of college, four years of medical school, three years of residency, and six years of full-time practice in the ER, I had to take another examination! This was 1989, in the early years of emergency medicine. Some of the physicians next to me had completed three years of training in one of the few certified EM Residency training programs, they qualified directly to take the certifying exam. The others were similar to me: physicians who had completed residency programs in another specialty (typically family practice or general surgery), then decided to make a career in the ER. It was a requirement for us to work full time in an ER for five years (referred to as the "Grandfather" track) before qualifying to take the EM Board Examination.

To become "Board Certified" by ABMS (The American Board of Medical Specialties) as a specialist in EM each physician would have to pass the Board Exams. ABEM (American Board of Emergency Medicine) was responsible for administering the Board Exam. The exam was two parts: a written exam, followed 9 to 12 months later by an oral exam. You had to pass the written exam in order to take the oral exam. After passing both exams you would be "Board Certified" in EM: tangible proof of education, training, and expertise in EM. Hospitals were looking to hire board certified EM physicians. Shortly, this would become a requirement in most ERs.

This was my first time with any sort of oral exam. The written exam was certainly challenging, but significantly less stressful. One could hardly become a physician if you weren't proficient at taking examinations. I was a disciplined and dedicated student, took many practice exams and routinely did well on the real thing. I passed the written board exam with flying colors. The oral exam would be a different story. With a young family and working full time I hadn't been able to take one of the few available courses in preparation. I was able to watch a few videos. I was confident about my medical knowledge and hoped I could answer questions well orally. There would be three examiners in each room. A presenter, who would present a clinical ER case and provide the questions for me to answer. A scorer, who would take notes and score my answers. Also, one observer, who's function I didn't really understand. There would be six rooms to go to, each with a different case presentation. Five cases would take up to 20 minutes each. One multiple case presentation would take up to 40 minutes.

The clock ticked to 1 PM and down the hall 20 physicians marched to each of our assigned rooms. I entered the room. In front of me was a long table. Three physician examiners sat straight and stoically behind the table; I stood in front. They looked at me, stone faced and serious. They checked my ID badge, and the exam started. The first case presentation was a 63-year-old man, agitated and pacing in an ER room. No one was with him. I started asking the patient's history. All the answers given to me were completely confusing. The "Patient" kept repeating nonsensical answers.

I realized the case was likely a patient with delirium, an uncommon and serious condition. Immediately I panicked. Hesitating and stammering, my mind went blank. I became clammy and started to sweat. I couldn't think of anything to do or ask. I described performing a non-focused general physical examination.

"What's the differential diagnosis?" the presenter asked.

All I could come up with was, "Agitation." That was a sign or symptom, certainly not an accurate diagnosis. I should have given a list of six or eight possibilities. Not knowing what to order, I asked for a huge array of blood and urine tests.

They said, "The laboratory was down, no results would be coming back." I asked for a CT head. They said it couldn't be performed, "The patient is too agitated." I asked for consultations, no specialists were available. I said I would admit the patient to the ICU. After a few more minutes of floundering around, the case ended. I left the room exhausted and defeated.

Heading back to the lobby after just a few steps, the light bulb turned on. Oh my goodness, I recognized this case. It was a presentation of DTs (Delirium Tremens) from severe alcohol withdrawal. Immediately the differential diagnosis jumped into my brain, specific tests to run, and medications to order. I wanted to turn around, go back, and give all the right answers. Of course, it was too late. I'd completely choked under pressure. I knew all about choking. I had played competitive tennis throughout high school and college. Everyone playing serious tennis matches has choked at one time or another. I certainly had.

Thoroughly demoralized, I limped into the lobby. I knew I flunked. What a waste! Oh well, the worst that would happen was paying another exam fee and returning next year. Pretty bad, but suddenly, somehow, I relaxed. The break would be 10 minutes. I gazed out the lobby window as other physicians returned from their exam rooms. We weren't allowed to talk to each other. Glancing at them I couldn't help noticing their demeanor. Most of them appeared devastated. Many were pale and perspiring, a few fighting back tears. I'd never seen such a group of depressed physicians. They were in much worse emotional shape than I was. It occurred to me to check if there were any windows that could open to the outside. I half wondered if someone might jump, to end this nightmare quickly. I felt much better and knew I couldn't do any worse. I decided to use the next five cases as practice and preparation for next time.

The 10-minute break passed quickly. We went to our next exam room, same set up and format. The presenter started the case. I listened carefully. Immediately I began asking appropriate questions to obtain the history. I verbally performed a relevant and focused PE. A straightforward differential diagnosis popped into my brain. The few important tests to request came to mind easily. The examiner reported the test results. The diagnosis was confirmed. I ordered treatment. The whole encounter lasted about 10 minutes. I was absolutely certain I nailed it. I walked back to the lobby. I was the first one back. When the other physicians returned, they looked even worse than before. Terrified, and moving slowly and stiffly, some were nearly catatonic. I felt badly for them, but there was nothing I could do.

The next four cases went extremely well, even the simultaneous multiple patient encounter. My responses were direct and confident. I answered quickly, pausing so the scorer could catch up on his note taking. I noticed the examiners looking at me strangely after I watched a hawk gliding by on an updraft outside the hotel room window. I was calm and comfortable, relaxed and breathing slowly. All the cases were challenging scenarios. Most were well described in the EM literature. I pointed out the pitfalls to avoid. I'd be ready next time.

Six weeks passed. An envelope from ABEM arrived in the mail. I opened it quickly, wanting to see how I'd performed overall. Shockingly, I passed! Had a great score too. How could that be? I could hardly believe it. There was absolutely no way, not after completely choking off that first case. Reading through the details, I discovered that for each examinee one of the five short cases would be thrown out. One of those cases would be practice for the examiners. Luckily, I hadn't known that fact while taking that oral exam. I doubt I would have relaxed. It certainly didn't matter now. I was Board Certified in Emergency Medicine.

Do You Believe In Miracles

It was about 3 AM on a bitter cold February night. The ER was
quiet. An 18-year-old man burst through the EMS doors hollering,
"Help! Help! My girlfriend's having a baby." The staff hesitated a
bit. Usually, these types of things are not an emergency, just
people panicking. I walked out the doors with him to his car. We
went to the front passenger side and opened the door.
"AAAAHHHH," loud screaming from a young woman. She was
throwing her head side to side in severe discomfort. She was semi-
reclined in the tilt back seat. I could see her gravid abdomen.
"AAAAHHHH," more loud screams.

The car interior was dimly lit. There was swelling between her
legs. I pulled the expandable waistline of her pants. There was an
infant head at the vaginal opening. The head was deeply purplish
black, severe cyanosis from a lack of oxygen. When the baby is
stuck in the birth canal the umbilical cord can be compressed and
not deliver enough oxygen. Also, the lungs cannot expand to
breathe. The infant's life was in critical danger. "We have to
deliver your baby now." The mother's only response was
continued screams. I had no idea how long the infant's head was
out, and the body stuck.

"Take a deep breath and push! Push!" I ordered. Screaming was
her only response. I felt the baby's neck. There was no nuchal cord
(umbilical cord wrapped around the neck). With gentle pulling on
the head nothing happened. I was concerned about shoulder
dystocia, where the infant's shoulder becomes caught behind the
mother's pubic bone and impairs delivery. I pulled harder and
pushed the head posteriorly. Out popped the anterior shoulder. I
put two fingers into the axilla and pulled, quickly delivering the

baby. The entire body was purplish black, severe discoloration. The baby made no effort to breathe. I palpated the umbilical cord and found pulsations. Hopefully this would provide circulation and oxygen to the infant. Placing the baby on the mother's chest I covered the infant with my lab coat. "Rub your baby." We needed to get the baby to our infant resuscitation warmer.

Leaning back, I stuck my head over the opened car door and motioned to Anne (the midnight shift RN) who was standing behind the glass entry door. She opened the door but didn't step outside. Not wanting to cause panic I politely asked, "Annie, would you quickly bring me a pair of scissors?"

Crossing her arms in front of her chest she said, "What do you need scissors for?"

I lost it. "Dammit! Go get the scissors!" I exploded. She ran back into the ER. I rubbed the infant vigorously. There was no coughing, crying or attempt to breathe. The baby remained a horrible purplish black color. The mother appeared stable and had stopped screaming. There was no meconium staining or serious vaginal bleeding. In a moment Anne arrived with scissors. I cut the cord. "Hold this end tight (mothers end), I'll send someone to help you get mom inside."

I gripped the umbilical cord and ran the infant to the neonatal warmer. By this time the entire staff was around. Simultaneously we rubbed and dried the infant with coarse towels and blew high flow oxygen towards the mouth and nose. I checked the heart rate, it was under 100, very dangerous. I started chest compressions and the respiratory therapist started ventilation with a tiny BVM (bag, valve, mask). BVM is a pliable bag with an oxygen line connected to a face mask. When the bag is compressed, it forces air and oxygen through the mask and into the patient. After 30 seconds we could see some respiratory effort. I rechecked the heartbeat. It was now 120. I stopped the compressions.

We kept drying, scrubbing, and giving oxygen. The infant started crying weakly, and some of the dark purplish color improved. I clamped the umbilical cord close to the infant and trimmed the end. A quick neonatal examination was normal, except for the severe acrocyanosis (purplish hands and feet). "It's a boy." I palpated the clavicles, nice and smooth. Likely not fractured with my pulling during delivery. After another two minutes the crying became stronger, and the infant's color improved. I estimated the APGAR scores (Appearance, Pulse, Grimace, Activity, and Respiration) scores - a test for how the baby tolerated the birthing process. At 1, 5, and 10 minutes the scores were: 2, 5 and 8. A score of 10 is the best, but 8 or 9 is good. The infant's prognosis was excellent.

I went to check on the mother, now in a hospital gown under a warm blanket in the room next door. She was 18 years old and doing well. The placenta had just been delivered and was intact. There was no active bleeding. Turns out this couple had no insurance and tried to have the baby at home. After many hours of labor, the pain became too intense, so they jumped in the car and drove to our ER. "We'll need to observe your baby for a while. There was a lot of cyanosis, that purple color. I think he will be fine because he has responded so quickly." The mother and child were transferred upstairs.

The RNs in the newborn nursery learned this young couple were planning to give their baby up for adoption but had yet to start the process. Our health care site was a small place where everyone knew everyone else. Those RNs knew Claire (an ER technician) and her husband had been trying to adopt a child for months. One RN called, was Claire working? By coincidence, Claire had just started her 7 AM shift. The parents wanted to meet her. Claire ran upstairs and became acquainted with the parents, additional meetings followed. The adoption agency was contacted, and the paperwork completed. Soon thereafter, Claire and her husband had a brand-new baby.

In the ER you never know what the day will bring.

Mistakes

They taught how to perform a thorough physical exam throughout medical school and polished those points during residency. I missed a key component. It took me ten years to figure it out. In the ER we do not have time to perform a complete physical exam on every patient. We do a "Focused" examination depending on the patient's chief complaint and history of present illness. This allows us to efficiently care for numerous ill and injured individuals. The "Key" component is that the physician must think about what to look for while doing each part of the physical exam. Following are some examples:

In pediatric patients with cough, it is important to consider pneumonia or asthma as possible causes. I recall many cases where I auscultated the lungs as "Clear" and yet the chest X-ray showed an obvious pneumonia. When I went back and listened carefully, I could hear the tell-tale "Rales" (tiny crackles) of pneumonia, e specially when listening at the very end of expiration. The same is true for wheezes in bronchospasm and asthma. One must listen carefully at the end of exhalation and think, "Are there wheezes?" at the same time. In patients with mild pneumonia or asthma, the sounds may only be present when the airways constrict during end of expiration.

In another case I admitted an elderly patient with sepsis (a serious infection). My skin exam was "Normal." No rashes or lesions. I couldn't find the source of the patient's infection. A short time later, the NP (nurse practitioner) called me about the badly infected sacral decubitus ulcer (a common skin wound on the sacrum due to pressure) she found during her admitting physical exam. The patient was weak, debilitated and confused so didn't complain about the bed sore or discomfort. The antibiotics were changed, and wound care started. The skin exam isn't complete until you roll the patient over and inspect the backside.

I saw a 67-year-old man with abdominal pain and fever. I found severe tenderness in the right upper quadrant and diagnosed acute cholecystitis (gallbladder infection). I called the chief surgical resident, ordered an US (ultrasound study), and wrote admitting orders. An hour later the surgeons were transferring my patient with an "AAA" (Abdominal Aortic Aneurysm) to the OR (Operating Room). An aneurysm is a diseased and dilated artery.

"What do you mean AAA?" I asked. They had seen him in Radiology, where the ultrasound scanner found gallstones, a thickened gallbladder wall and an eight-centimeter (over three inch) AAA. I stopped the cart in the hallway and gently palpated the patient's abdomen just below the umbilicus. In the midline was a large pulsatile mass, the AAA. I had completely missed it by not finishing my abdominal exam. In the OR (operating room) they removed the infected gallbladder. They planned to repair the AAA in a few days. There were two critical diagnoses, not just one. I stopped looking too soon.

I saw a 60-year-old man with a sudden onset of abdominal pain and vomiting. On my physical exam his abdomen was distended, had no scars, was distended, and had mild diffuse tenderness. I found no hernia. The abdominal X-ray confirmed a SBO (small bowel obstruction). I consulted general surgery. After they saw the patient, they asked me to reduce the incarcerated hernia (trapped bowel in the abdominal wall). I said I didn't find any hernia. They said, "Check the umbilicus." Sure enough, on my repeat exam there was a small, tender mass near the belly button. I had only checked the inguinal region for hernias. I didn't carefully examine the umbilicus. Pretty embarrassing. Hernias often occur in scars and near the umbilicus, not just the groin.

Early in my career there were quite a few times I diagnosed anemia (low hemoglobin or red blood cell count) after getting the laboratory tests back. I had not expected anemia because I had failed to note the patient's pale skin, conjunctiva, and nail beds. This occurred at least five times and convinced me that I don't always learn from my mistakes. In fact, I kept repeating the same mistake. It's easy to learn from mistakes that have immediate severe consequences (think placing your fingers on a hot stove), and often difficult otherwise.

I was supervising Casey, a PA (physician assistant) who had many years of experience. She presented an 84-year-old-man to me who complained of left buttock pain radiating down the left leg. She felt the diagnosis was sciatica or a bulging disc since there was weakness of the left leg. On my physical examination the left leg was cool, pale and had no palpable pedal (foot) pulses. We consulted vascular surgery STAT (from the Latin word statim, meaning immediately). The patient had a clot removed from his left femoral artery. If you do not think of a diagnosis, it is difficult to perform the correct "Focused" exam (if you think of a blocked blood supply, then you check the pulses carefully).

The patient's history of the present illness strongly suggests the diagnosis in 80 to 90 percent of cases presenting to the ER. The physician must keep in mind the possible diagnoses from this history while performing the physical exam. If pneumonia is a possibility, then the focus is on the respiratory rate, the oxygen measurement and careful lung auscultation. If asthma is a possibility, then one must listen carefully for wheezes and a prolonged expiration (the narrowed airways don't allow smooth exhalation of inspired air). The physical findings help confirm or rule out the diagnostic possibilities considered from the patient history.

"My lymph nodes are swollen," Melissa said anxiously. She was 15-years-old, brought to the ER by her concerned mother. Melissa had been in excellent health until two months prior when she noticed swelling on the right side of her face. It was mildly tender and gradually increased in size. She went to her family doctor who diagnosed a swollen preauricular (in front of the ear) lymph node. Lab tests were normal, negative for strep and mono. Her doctor prescribed cephalexin (an antibiotic) for 10 days for a possible infection. There was no improvement, and she was referred to a plastic surgeon for biopsy. The biopsy showed nonspecific inflammation.

In the last few days Melissa noticed two non-tender swollen lumps on the right side of her neck. Her mother was worried about swollen lymph nodes, "Something else might be going on," (she didn't say the word cancer in front of her daughter). There were no other symptoms. No fever, fatigue, bug or tick bites, rash, jaundice, or recent infections. She had received routine childhood immunizations.

On the physical exam I paid particular attention to palpating her liver, spleen, and lymph nodes. The only abnormalities I could find were two small, firm, mobile, nontender lymph nodes on the right side of her neck, and the healing incision secondary to the biopsy in front of her ear. All else was completely normal. Puzzled, I sent off routine lab tests. These were not likely to be helpful. I was hoping to reassure Melissa and her mother and needed to make a diagnosis. With no hepatosplenomegaly and no adenopathy (other swollen lymph nodes) lymphoma, leukemia or cancer were unlikely. The blood tests returned normal. She would have to follow up with Hem / Onc (Hematology / Oncology) for further testing.

I was typing up discharge instructions for "Lymphadenopathy" when a thought occurred to me. Returning to the patient's room I asked Melissa and her mother, "In the last six months did you get a cat?" They seemed a bit surprised at the question.

"Yes," they replied.

"Was it a kitten?"

"Yes."

"Were you scratched?"

"Yes, when playing with the kitten I got little scratches on the right hand and shoulder."

"You have cat scratch disease," I pronounced. "It's a bacterial infection (Bartonella henselae). It's transmitted from cats, especially kittens. Most people improve without treatment, but in your case, we'll prescribe a different antibiotic. Your lymph nodes will gradually return to normal." Both Melissa and her mother were relieved and smiled for the first time, happy to have a benign diagnosis. I followed up about a month later. The swelling disappeared.

If a physician doesn't know the condition or doesn't think of it (cat scratch disease) it is nearly impossible to diagnose it. In this case, Melissa had seen two doctors. She underwent numerous unnecessary tests, and a biopsy. I nearly missed the diagnosis as well. I was too concerned and anchored on the possibility of cancer. It wasn't until I considered the many causes of lymphadenopathy (while preparing the discharge instructions). Best to keep an open mind.

———————————

It was one of those nights. Complete chaos. The hospital wards were full, the ER was packed. Every hallway was lined with patients on carts awaiting admission (to unavailable inpatient beds). I had over 24 names on my patient list, a few were critically ill.

Mrs. Sullivan was brought in by her daughters. She was 86-years-old with a history of dementia, hypertension, heart failure, recurrent UTIs (urinary tract infections), and an allergy to PCN (penicillin). She developed a fever, weakness, and could no longer walk. There was no cough, vomiting, fall or trauma. Her VS: temp of 101, RR (respiratory rate) 24, HR (heart rate) 124, and BP 128 / 80, and pulse ox of 95 %. She was dehydrated with dry lips and oral mucous membranes. I couldn't find any source of infection on physical examination. We rolled her over to check for decubiti, there were none.

The diagnosis was sepsis, an infection spreading through Mrs. Sullivan. She needed IV fluids and antibiotics. If started early (before hypotension or shock), her prognosis was good. Another UTI was the likely cause. I asked her RN Sheryl, "Can you test the urine with a dipstick to check for WBCs when you do the bladder catheterization? If positive, it would bear a clear sign of an infection. Let me know the results, and I'll pick the antibiotics. Thanks."

I went to my desk and entered routine orders for sepsis. I reviewed the results for two other patients and prepared their discharge instructions. They had been in the ER for over four hours. I wanted to get them on their way, and to open their rooms for additional patients from the waiting room. Another patient needed a central IV line, the procedure often takes 20 or 30 minutes. I needed to do that shortly.

After discharging the two patients I was walking past the nurses' station to begin the central line. Sheryl said, "Dr. Thomson, I did the urine dipstick. It was strongly positive for WBCs."

"That confirms urosepsis," I said. "Start 3 grams of unasyn and 120 mg of gentamicin for Mrs. Sullivan. I'll put the orders in after

I start the central line. Thanks." I finished the central line and went back to my desk and documented the procedure.

I opened Mrs. Sullivan's medical record to enter the antibiotic orders. Immediately I saw Allergies: penicillin. Uh oh. I ran to her room. An empty bag of unasyn (a type of penicillin) was hanging on her IV pole. I examined Mrs. Sullivan. No allergic reaction, no hives, rash, wheezing or hypotension. What good fortune. I found Sheryl. "Did you know Mrs. Sullivan had an allergy to penicillin listed on her chart?"

"I saw that," she replied. "But I know that most patients aren't truly allergic, and you always check it out. So, I overrode the pyxis (computer controlled locked medication cabinet) allergy block."

"Sheryl, thanks for your confidence in me, but be careful. You must double check. I was so busy I forgot about her allergies and didn't check with her family. Keep a close eye on her for the next hour." Most severe allergic reactions start within 30 minutes.

How had I made such a clear mistake? In retrospect a few things were obvious. I was multitasking. I was in a hurry. I had a critical (distracting) task looming. I gave a verbal order. Entering orders directly in the patient's medical record is much safer; the allergy listing is directly in front of you. I made a note to discuss nursing and pharmacy review of physician orders at the next staff meeting, to ensure appropriate double checking. It was only luck that the patient didn't have an allergic reaction. It easily could have been life threatening.

If you think that you are a good multitasker, you are making an error. Add in a chaotic ER environment, interruptions, stress, fatigue, circadian rhythm changes, and complex decision making then critical mistakes result. If not, then you are early in your career or not human. It is difficult to learn from your mistakes, and easy to keep repeating them. Looking in the mirror and admitting I made a mistake was the hard part (and the necessary first step).

Don't Panic

Dr. Thomson! Dr. Thomson!!" Mary the triage RN screamed as she ran into the ER with a large emesis basin. Inside was a bright pink, 14 inch long, thumb sized diameter worm. It was writhing vigorously like an excited snake.

"Where did you get that?" I asked.

"A girl at triage just vomited it up! She came in complaining of nausea over the past few days and thought she might throw up. She started retching, so I handed her a basin and out came that snake! She says she's going to vomit again. It's like The Exorcist."

Mary was an excellent nurse and loved the drama and chaos of the ER. Normally imperturbable, she slowly caught her breath. I explained that this was a common human parasitic worm, Ascaris lumbricoides which infects over one of every six people on the planet. I had seen one in a specimen jar at Kalamazoo College, vomited up by a student returning from foreign study. It was kept in a collection with many other similar human parasites, all brought to campus by traveling students.

Shelly, the now trembling young patient was brought to an exam room. She had been on a mission to Africa and returned one week before. Besides her GI (gastrointestinal) upset there were no other symptoms. Her physical examination was normal. She began retching again. Out of her mouth came an identical writhing worm. Watching a live object exiting the oral cavity easily allows observers to believe that someone could be possessed. (They are, by a human parasite). We sent one specimen to pathology for confirmation. I diagnosed Ascaris infection and prescribed mebendazole, an antiparasitic medication. The drug is effective and has few side effects. I reassured Shelly and recommended follow up in two weeks to ensure resolution.

———————————

On a sunny July afternoon, a 30-year-old woman in a swimsuit presented to the ER with, "A fly went in my ear." She had been sunbathing and felt a fly land near her right ear. After brushing it off with her hand it landed again a few minutes later. This time when she brushed it away, it went down into her ear canal. I had seen this a few times before and was puzzled by her calm appearance. Every previous patient with a fly stuck in the ear canal was anxious and episodically nearly hysterical with discomfort. When a fly buzzes next to the tympanic membrane (ear drum) the vibration and loud sound is intolerable. Flies often buzz every minute or two when deep in the ear canal. This woman was sitting peacefully in our ENT (ear, nose, and throat) chair. She denied any buzzing sounds.

I checked her left ear canal and ear drum: perfectly normal. Looking through the otoscope down the right ear canal I saw a black object with at least two black legs next to the tympanic membrane. It was partially obscured by wax and the normal slight curve in the ear canal. There was no movement or buzzing. "I see an insect in your ear canal. I'll put in a few drops of mineral oil. In a minute the insect will drown and be easier to remove."

She was placed in a semi fowler position (reclining about 40 degrees) in the ENT chair. I turned her head to the left, pulled up and back on her ear to straighten the ear canal, and dripped in eight drops of mineral oil. Three seconds passed. An insect appeared at the opening of the ear canal. Suddenly a fat, hairy spider jumped onto my left wrist. Reflexly, I jerked my hand back, howled "Yeeeooooww," and watched the spider fly vertically about three feet. Amazingly, the spider dropped straight back down onto the patient's cheek, and immediately scurried back down into her ear canal! Two seconds passed. The large black spider reappeared and cautiously crawled down her cheek. I quickly brushed it off to the floor. It crawled towards the door but met its end as I stomped it three times with my foot.

Meanwhile the patient remained motionless, seemingly oblivious to my panicked treatment efforts. It was the first time I screamed in the ER. Open fractured bones, gunshot wounds, purulent abscess material, and spurting blood had never surprised me like that ugly spider. I apologized to the young woman, but she remained unconcerned. "Be careful," I joked. "In about two weeks about 100 baby spiders might crawl out."

Now she seemed worried, "Really?"

"No chance of that," I replied. "But we'll irrigate your ear canal thoroughly. Just to be sure."

It Just Popped In There

A 37-year-old woman was placed into room 11. I introduced myself and said, "Tell me what happened." She anxiously described numerous symptoms. "Over the last few days my legs seem tingly, numb, and my muscles ache. It's hard to walk. I feel weak." There was no fever, fall, trauma, back pain, or trouble urinating. She didn't think she could be pregnant. The LMP (last menstrual period) was 10 days ago. The ROS (review of systems) was a different story: headaches, tinnitus, dizziness, trouble swallowing, heartburn, chest pain, shortness of breath, bloating, gas, diarrhea, constipation. The more time I spent the more symptoms she described. It was difficult to sort through them all. Her exam was unremarkable. She had good grip strength, good plantar flexion and extension, no muscle tenderness, no fasciculations or tremors. The thyroid gland was palpably normal. I couldn't find anything.

I returned to my desk to write orders. I was totally stumped. There was a bewildering number of seemingly unrelated symptoms. In her case the diagnosis was likely to be anxiety, stress, or hypochondriasis. Many of those patients have frequent visits to the ER or their PCP. She didn't. In fact, this was her first time to the ER. I couldn't think of where to start.

Just then Elaine (a very experienced RN who had seen this patient in triage) stopped by and asked, "What did you think of the woman I put into room 11?"

"Absolutely no idea," I replied, "I can't even think of what tests to order."

"Well," she said, "I once saw a patient like her, years ago on the hospital ward. Do you know what she had?"

"Not a clue. What?" I inquired.

"Guillain-Barre," Elaine stated matter of factly.

Oh my goodness. That diagnosis would fit beautifully. Guillain-Barre was a rare syndrome. It was thought to be an inflammatory process following a gastrointestinal or respiratory infection. It was extremely difficult to diagnose in its early stages due to a myriad number of mild symptoms and minimal signs on exam. One of the few reliable findings were markedly diminished or absent DTRs (deep tendon reflexes) which I had failed to examine. Blood tests are normal. Spinal fluid protein was reliably elevated.

I immediately strolled back to room 11 and tapped her biceps, triceps, patellar, and Achilles tendons. All were significantly diminished. Guianne-Barre jumped to the top of the list of likely possibilities. Careful observation of her gait revealed cautious, unsteady steps. These subtle abnormal physical exam findings were present (if the physician knew what to look for). The panel of lab tests returned normal. The patient agreed to a lumbar puncture to obtain spinal fluid. Sure enough, the protein level was markedly elevated.

I paged the admitting hospital physician. He accepted the patient to his service but was skeptical about the diagnosis. The elevated spinal fluid test convinced him that something serious was going on, and that she needed neurologic consultation and additional evaluation. The next day he called me back. The neurologist had seen the patient and agreed that Guillain-Barre was likely. More importantly, the patient rapidly developed serious generalized weakness, respiratory failure, and required intubation. He was amazed that I considered the diagnosis and wanted to know how I'd even thought of it. I told him the whole story about how I was dumbfounded until Elaine picked it right off. She deserved all the credit.

Over the next two weeks the patient stabilized, then improved and was taken off the ventilator. Numerous residents and attending physicians rotated care throughout her hospital stay. I kept getting compliments about my diagnostic acumen. After the third or fourth time I tired of reciting the long "Elaine RN" story. So, when I heard again, "How did your brain even think of it?"

I would exclaim, "I don't know. It just popped in there!"

Munchausen's Syndrome

Munchausen's Syndrome is a psychological disorder where the patient pretends to be ill, so that people care for them, and they receive lots of attention. Most ERs have patients that present frequently, and a rare one or two that come in 50 or more times a year. EMTALA (Emergency Medical Treatment and Labor Act) is a federal law that requires anyone coming to the ER to be stabilized and treated. Hospitals receiving funds from Medicare are required to perform a "Screening medical examination" on every patient that presents to the ER and must ensure there is no emergency. Medicare is usually the largest payer of medical bills. The result is we must see all comers. The "Over 50 Club" are patients that are often homeless, addicted to drugs / alcohol or have Munchausen's syndrome.

One 44-year-old man was a homeless patient with chronic severe alcoholism. During the colder months he would present to our ER two to three times per week. His preferred method was to walk to the nearest road and lay down near the curb. Someone in a passing car would call EMS. Within minutes an EMS unit would arrive and immediately transport him to our ER. At first, he received customary care. He would be placed directly in a private room, given a gown and a warm blanket. His usual chief complaint was either chest pain or, "I'm too drunk."

He had occasionally been admitted to the hospital and underwent thorough evaluations. Besides the alcohol dependency disorder, we could never identify any other significant pathology. Of course, after a few weeks we got tired of this. We had special departmental meetings including IM (Internal Medicine), Psychiatry, and Social Work. Nothing helped. He was transferred a few times to an inpatient substance abuse treatment center. This failed. They would refuse to readmit him. Psychiatry prescribed medication, he didn't take it. He was often discharged to a homeless shelter. If the weather was poor, we knew we would see him again soon.

Another sad case was Mary, a 26-year-old woman who would present frequently to our Jackson ER with complaints of abdominal pain. This happened about 50 times over 12 years. The type, severity, duration of pain and accompanying symptoms would vary. Mary would wince convincingly upon palpation of her abdomen. Every conceivable blood and urine test had been ordered, as well as multiple US (Ultrasound) and CAT scans. She'd been admitted numerous times and underwent exploratory surgery twice. Nothing serious was ever diagnosed. Over the many years she was seen by multiple ER physicians.

One day it was my turn. I went to her room and started my history and exam. She appeared calm and in no distress. She admitted to being evaluated a couple of times in the past for abdominal pain and had surgery many years previously. There was a linear, midline scar above the umbilicus, consistent with exploratory surgery. Upon palpation of the abdomen, she seemed extremely tender in the RUQ (right upper quadrant). I indicated that the nurses would set her up for a pelvic exam.

I went to place some routine orders. Our computer system had recently been upgraded. It was now possible to retrieve radiology studies including US and CT scan results from the last six years. I found results of numerous abdominal and pelvic US examinations; all were normal. There were multiple CT scans of the abdomen and pelvis, most with IV contrast. Again, all were normal. I counted the CT scans: 16. I manually retrieved her entire radiology file and found seven additional scans. This young woman had 23 CT scans of her abdomen and pelvis. This was a phenomenally high amount of radiation exposure. I couldn't imagine her risk of cancer. Our ER was busy, seeing about 80,000 patients per year. Our physician group had more than 60 physicians. Over the 12 years only a few saw her more than once.

I returned to her room and repeated my exam. The only abnormality was wincing convincingly with abdominal palpation. I sat down for a lengthy discussion. She was totally unconcerned about any risks from radiation, or any risk of cancer. She became upset when I indicated that no tests would be run. No blood or urine tests, no X-rays, no US, and no CT scan. I asked her to follow up with her PCP and indicated that her PCP would receive a copy of my dictated ER note. If she developed new symptoms she could return to the ER. She should avoid future radiation if possible. She should let anyone know if tests were being ordered to review her previous results. I also informed her that I was putting a computer "Red Flag" into her medical record. This was an electronic notation that would pop up when medical providers were starting to order any radiological study. She was discharged without any tests, extremely unhappy. My efforts would likely have little effect on her behavior. Even with intensive therapy, patients with Munchausen's syndrome seldom change their behavior. Many patients often change their PCP or preferred ER.

April was 50-years-old. She would come in one or two times each week. Nearly always complaining of chest pain, so she wouldn't have to wait for an ER bed. She would be whisked back for a quick ECG (electrocardiogram). After 10 or 20 visits, if the ECG was normal, she would be placed back into the waiting room. After a few more visits, we dispensed with the ECG. April was a quick learner and soon developed other chief complaints. Many were potentially serious: sudden onset of severe headache, vomiting blood or blood in her stool; and swollen legs, "Like when I had a blood clot."

April had been admitted numerous times. No significant pathology was ever identified. Reviewing her chart one day I found numerous CT scans, both abdominal and chest. She'd had MRIs (magnetic resonance imaging) of the head and spine, upper and lower gastrointestinal endoscopy, and more than one cardiac echo and stress test. All the tests were normal. She did have a few stable medical problems: mild hypertension, obesity, and elevated cholesterol. We never found anything serious. Psychiatric consultation confirmed our suspicion of Munchausen syndrome. Despite our best efforts (referrals to PCP, Psychiatry, Social work) April continued to return frequently to our ER.

One particularly busy day she came in and was seen by a new triage nurse. The young RN was starting to bring her back to our ECG area when a more experienced nurse glanced up. Catching her in mid stride, she turned April around and walked her straight back to the waiting room. The area was packed with about 10 stable patients waiting for an ER bed, along with 20 to 30 family members and friends.

After a few minutes there was some commotion. Cries of "Help! Help! A lady is having a seizure." The panicked triage nurse ran back into the ER calling for assistance, "Someone is having a seizure." At that very moment I was walking past the entrance door. I quickly went into the waiting room and examined the seizing patient, and immediately recognized April (having cared for her on over 25 occasions). I paused briefly then shouted, "April! Quit faking! We're not taking you into the back."

Everyone in the waiting room was aghast, staring in total silence, completely stunned. First, there was a seizing patient. Second, at the exasperated physician yelling at the patient who was in apparent severe distress. Third, a moment later the seizure miraculously stopped! Then, April crawled up off the floor, sat in the nearest chair, bowed her head and murmured, "OK."

A 33-year-old woman with a history of Munchausen's syndrome had been seen many times by her PCP and in the ER. I had treated her a few times. She would present with symptoms of an infection, and often receive a Rx (Prescription) for an antibiotic. This ER presentation was markedly different. Her nurse came and asked me to see the patient immediately.

"She has the worst case of diarrhea I've ever seen. It's just pouring out of her. I'll bet its C diff."

The patient was pale, cool, clammy, tachycardic and hypotensive. The only other abnormality was her massive liquid stool output. I agreed, "Likely C diff."

Clostridium difficile diarrhea results from disruption of normal healthy bacteria in the colon, often due to antibiotic use. C diff can be strongly suspected in the ER due to its green color, watery consistency, and characteristic foul odor. Most young patients with C diff recover, but in older debilitated patients it can be fatal. The nurses started two large bore IV lines and gave a bolus of fluid and sent routine blood work. The laboratory tests returned with critical electrolyte and kidney function abnormalities. Her HR and BP improved marginally. She was critically ill. I inserted a central IV line, gave more IV fluids, and admitted her to the ICU.

A week later the Intensivist (ICU doctor) called and gave me a report, "Remember that patient with C diff?

"Uh oh. Yes," I replied, suspecting bad news was coming.

"She died this morning. Her course in the ICU was stormy. The diarrhea wouldn't stop. The surgeons resected (surgically removed) her colon. She developed septic shock and died." This was horrible. A perfectly healthy 33-year-old woman dying from unnecessary antibiotics. I sat in silence, reflecting on the senseless tragedy.

It was well recognized that antibiotics were overly prescribed. We tried to limit their use, but many patients were insistent. I had gotten a few complaints from patients with a likely viral infection who I did not prescribe antibiotics for. They went to their family doctor for a Rx (prescription). Then I would receive an angry complaint. "I got better in a few days. I'm not paying your bill." The easiest thing to do was to give in and write a Rx. In fact, I had given an antibiotic to this woman in the not-too-distant past. Knowing that I may have contributed to her death was especially troubling. Did my Rx precipitate her diarrhea and lead to her death?

One of the first things taught in medical school is a Latin phrase "Primum non nocere," "First do no harm." It is part of the Hippocratic Oath, an ancient ethical oath. Perhaps 6,000 years old, known from Greek medical textbooks. I resolved to not write prescriptions because the patient wanted medication, but only when indicated and the benefits outweigh the risks.

Night Shifts

The first 10 years of my career I worked four 12-hour day shifts, followed by four days off, followed by four 12-hour night shifts, and then again four days off. It was brutal. There were four full time physicians, none of us wanted to work all night shifts. We had to rotate. The fatigue from sleep deprivation was terrible. There are numerous studies about night shift work. It takes two days to recover after working a midnight shift, eight to recover after four midnight shifts. One solution is to work straight night shifts for a long period of time and keep the same sleep pattern. Of course, your family is likely not in this pattern.

These studies found many health problems associated with rotating night shift work: decreased mental performance, decreased memory, errors, depression, diabetes, obesity, reflux, ulcers, and heart disease. With lack of sleep and the resulting extreme fatigue I was often irritable and short tempered. Throw in a particularly busy day in the ER and I could be extremely difficult to live with.

One low point as a physician occurred when I began to evaluate a man with chest pain. Jane, an ER tech, handed me his ECG. There were changes consistent with an AMI (acute myocardial infarction / heart attack). Upon entering the room, it was obvious the patient was in serious distress. He was anxious, pale, clammy, and profusely diaphoretic. Angry, I turned to Jane and said, "Why didn't you come and get me before the ECG? I need to see patients like this immediately!" I took care of the patient, sent him to the cardiac Cath (Catheter) lab, and forgot about my outburst.

Not even one month later, I was at my desk entering orders. It was a particularly busy day. Jane interrupted me and asked, "Can you come to room 1 and see a patient with chest pain?" I signed the orders, then quickly went to room 1. There was a middle-aged man complaining of severe substernal chest pain. He was short of breath, vomiting, and in obvious discomfort. "Where's his ECG," I demanded.

The nurses were starting an IV and hooking the patient up to monitors. "We didn't get it yet," Jane answered softly.

I was upset and said, "I thought our protocol was to get the ECG first." Jane looked surprised and flustered, almost bursting into tears. She left the room. The nurses obtained an ECG quickly. There were some minor changes, but no heart attack. The patient was stable and after a short while he was admitted.

Towards the end of my shift, Marsha (an RN caring for the patient) came into the physician work room. "Can I talk with you for a minute?" she asked. We went down the hall to the break room. Marsha was one of the most experienced nurses, compassionate and altruistic. We'd worked together for many years. She taught me a great deal about the practice of medicine, just by her example.

"Dr. Thomson, I heard what you said to Jane. You're right, getting the ECG first is the protocol. But I was here a month ago and I heard you say just the opposite. You needed to see the sick patients right away and not wait until after the ECG was done. Jane was just doing what you requested. You can't have it both ways. We'll do whatever you decide. Worse yet, you shouldn't talk to Jane like that. You were almost yelling at her."

"Oh boy, I don't know why I am so short tempered. I'd like to blame it on sleep deprivation, but that's just an excuse. Thanks for telling me."

I found Jane and apologized. She graciously accepted. I was supposed to be a leader of the department, and probably was on my good days. I needed to be a good leader every day.

I realized I was similarly irritable at home with my wife and children. I looked in the mirror and vowed to change. One of my few regrets about a career in EM was having to work so many midnights, weekends, and holidays. I am certain my family suffered. Within a few years I was able to decrease the number of night shifts to three per month. When I turned 55, I was able to avoid all night shifts (our group added extra compensation to physicians willing to staff the overnight hours). Avoiding those circadian rhythm changes added years to my career.

––––––––––––––––

In the first 10 years, after midnight we would typically see only three or four patients until about 7 AM. Staffing was light, usually the physician, one RN, one RT (respiratory therapist), one laboratory technician, and one X-ray technician. Over the years you'd get to know your coworkers well.

In radiology we had plain X-ray films and a CT scanner for head imaging only. All films would be brought to the emergency department and initially be read by the emergency physician. The radiologist would read the studies the next morning and dictate their final report. We kept a log of all the patients and our initial readings to compare with the final radiology report. Any discrepancies would be reviewed, and patients contacted as necessary. After a few years my readings improved, and there were fewer discrepancies. Nan the full-time radiology technician, was extremely sharp. If she realized that special views would be important, she would quickly take them. When returning the patient and films to the ER she would let me know to add the additional orders. It was an efficient system.

One night about 1 AM, I was evaluating a patient. He was sitting on a bench close to the radiology viewing box. He'd injured his left ankle playing basketball and couldn't bear any weight. Upon examination he had significant localized tenderness over the lateral malleolus. Our triage nurse had ordered the X-rays. They were up on the view box ready for my interpretation. I couldn't see a fracture.

I started to explain to the patient: "You likely have a severe sprain. We will provide you ....," I was interrupted by someone clearing their throat. I started giving instructions again. Another throat clearing, this time louder. Glancing over, I saw Nan. With brief head tilts she indicated I should look back at the view box. I did. Still no fracture or dislocation was evident. Puzzled, I asked, "What's up Nan?"

"Check the lateral view," she advised.

Upon careful inspection of the lateral view, I could easily see the fractured distal fibula. It was invisible on the AP view. But no question, there it was on the lateral. I backtracked and showed the patient his fractured ankle. We'll put on a temporary plaster splint, give you some crutches, and have you follow up with the orthopedist.

After the patient left, Nan and the other staff could hardly contain their laughter.

"You're a doofus," she exclaimed.

"What are you talking about?"

"How many years have we been working together?" she asked.

"About 8 to 10 years I'd guess."

"Well, haven't you noticed? Sometimes I place the films on the view box and other times the films are in the envelope on the shelf beneath it," she pointed out.

"Sure," I replied.

"Well," she said, laughing, "Anytime I see a fracture, the X-rays are up on the view box. When the X-rays are normal, they're inside the envelope." Was I a slow learner! For years, I knew Nan was excellent at interpreting films. I had wondered about the pattern but never figured out the obvious.

_____

I was on my fourth night shift in a row, at 5 AM I was completely exhausted. The ER had only one patient, awaiting transfer to an inpatient room. I told the staff I was going to lay down in the on-call room. At some point I had the telephone in my ear, and someone was screaming, "Dr. Thomson! Wake Up! I need you to come see this patient immediately." I was still groggy, "Ok, ok, I'm on my way."

I walked to the ER. A 72-year-old man had arrived via EMS. He was lethargic, hyperventilating and smelled of ketones (a sweet, fruity odor). He had a long history of insulin dependent diabetes, peripheral neuropathy, hypertension, and heart disease. According to his wife he was feeling poorly for a day or two. His blood sugars were running high, and they planned on calling his doctor the next morning. He woke up confused and could not get out of bed, so she called 911. I was examining him as his wife relayed the history. He was in critical condition, severely dehydrated, tachycardic and hypotensive. With the fruity odor this was likely DKA (diabetic ketoacidosis) a common life-threatening condition in brittle diabetics.

His exam wasn't remarkable except for his left leg. It was cold and pale, mottled blue and red, and there were no palpable pulses. When I palpated his quadriceps muscle my four fingers left deep indentations, like I had pressed into cookie dough. I had never seen that before. We started the standard care and treatment for DKA, notified the ICU of the upcoming admission, and called the vascular surgeon, Dr. Jenson. I presented the case: "I think he's clotted off his left Iliac or Femoral artery. There are unusual depressions in the muscles of his cold left leg when I with my fingers."

Dr. Jenson replied, "That is the "Dough" sign. It's due to necrotic (dead) muscle. It's likely the leg is not salvageable. Admit him to the ICU. I'll come right in to examine him." The patient was transferred shortly to the ICU. His prognosis was grave.

I signed out to the oncoming day shift physician, then asked the nurses, "Who was yelling at me on the phone?"

Linda said, "I was." She related that when EMS arrived, she found the left leg to be ice cold. She immediately called me to come and see the patient and could tell that I wasn't fully awake. "I kept telling you that he was in bad shape and that his leg was cold. All you kept repeating was, "Put a blanket on it." After the third or fourth time, I was about to walk down the hall and knock on the door but yelled instead."

I had absolutely no recollection of the initial conversation. I was concerned. I struggled to think clearly at times (with the circadian rhythm changes, lack of sleep, and severe fatigue). I wondered how often I answered the phone and gave advice without being alert. That was the last time I attempted to sleep during night shifts.

Tragedy

"EMS Alpha 127 calling, how do you read?"

"Loud and clear," our charge nurse replied.

"We're en route with a two-year-old in full arrest. We're performing CPR (CardioPulmonary Resuscitation with chest compressions). Arrival time is four minutes."

"What are the VS?" we asked, wanting confirmation.

"Full arrest, unresponsive, apneic (no breathing), and no pulse. The HR monitor is flatline (no electrical activity). We are performing BVM and CPR and are unable to obtain IV access or intubate."

The EMS radio was at our main nurses' station, the physician work room just behind. I walked a few steps to Room 1, immediately joined by the charge nurse, another RN and two techs, the respiratory therapist and an X-ray tech were on the way. We pulled the peds crash cart to the bedside and opened it up.

The voices of my staff were high pitched, tense, frantic. Critically ill patients are seen daily in the ER. Death and dying patients are common events, fortunately quite rare in infants and children. In this pediatric case, everyone was anxious, waiting with dreaded anticipation. We had just a minute or two to prepare. I needed the team to be calm and to concentrate on the coming tasks. "Look, we'll check the monitor first. If it is flatline, the heart has completely stopped. The chance for a successful resuscitation is almost zero. But we're going to follow the PALS (Pediatric Advanced Life Support) protocol." In children it takes many minutes without oxygen for the heart to stop completely (flatline on the heart monitor). By that time, the brain is already dead.

The EMS unit arrived and rushed the child in. We checked the heart monitor in multiple leads, all flatline. Chest compressions were continued. The nurses attempted IV access. I was able to intubate the child without difficulty. Still unable to obtain an IV line I used a drill to place an IO (Intraosseous) line into the right proximal tibia. Multiple doses of epinephrine and bicarb were given, all without response. The history from the paramedics was that the parents had left for work. The babysitter had placed the child in a crib for its morning nap. After an hour or so the sitter went to check on the child. The infant was blue and unresponsive, hanging in a corner of the crib. He was wearing a hooded sweatshirt and the cord had somehow looped around a corner post and the lower part caught around the child's neck.

The babysitter called 911 and started chest compressions. Upon arrival EMS found the child unresponsive and flatline. There was never any response to their resuscitation efforts. The parents had been contacted and were on their way to the ER. They would arrive in about 30 minutes. We ran out of options. The child remained flatline. About 60 minutes had passed from the 911 call. There was no hope. I called the code. Certainly, the team was ready to go on. Perhaps until the parents arrived, to show them the heroic measures. No, I decided we were finished. I pronounced the little boy dead. His name was Nathan. I thanked the team. They were silent, most crying, gloom everywhere.

"I'll speak to the parents. Put them in the family room when they arrive." It's difficult to know how and when to break this tragic news to the family. They had been told there had been an "emergency" during his nap, and that he was brought by ambulance to the ER. If the patient has already been pronounced dead and the family over 30 to 60 minutes away, I would often tell them over the phone. Better not to have the acutely stressed family racing long distances to the ER (which might result in an accident). In this case, I would be telling the parents directly.

When hearing about the sudden death of a loved one there is typically a tremendous grief spike. With some warning and preparation for bad news one might lessen the severity of this painful spike a bit. Much of what is said before and after hearing horrible news is forgotten, so best not to say too much. Also, you must use the word "died" or "dead." If you are not clear (patient is gone, has passed, didn't make it, etc) there is often significant confusion. Of course, the family is hoping their loved one hasn't died.

"Dr. Thomson, the parents are here. We put them in the family room." I tapped on the door and entered. There was a young couple, obviously concerned and worried. They were silent and looked apprehensive. Taken directly to a quiet separate room and closing the door made them suspect bad news was coming. I sat down and introduced myself, and confirmed they were mother and father. This was their only child.

"Your babysitter put Nathan down for his nap. When she went to check on him, she found the sweatshirt cord caught around a corner post and his neck. He wasn't breathing so she called 911 and started chest compressions. The paramedics found the heart was stopped and brought him to the ER. We performed resuscitation and used all of our medications, but we couldn't restart the heart. I just pronounced him dead." There was a brief pause. The mother looked down, tears running silently. Dad wailed painfully. He too bowed his head and slumped to his wife. I sat quietly, waiting. After some time, I spoke softly. "I am so sorry. You'll likely have questions for me. I'll leave you alone for a few minutes. I'll come back and we can go see him shortly."

For most family members viewing the deceased body is important. It is frightening and difficult but helps the grieving process. Looking over the unresponsive body, and touching or holding a pale, cold hand confirms the death of their loved one in ways that words cannot.

The parents followed me into Room 1. I brought them to the bedside. Lifting a hand demonstrating, I told them it was certainly okay to hold their child. The father asked, "How do you think this happened?" I told them I'd read about some rare cases. It was likely he had tried to climb out of the crib and accidentally hooked the hood drawstring around the corner post. If he fell, the string could easily strangle his neck and prevent him from making any sound. They bent forward, their heads against the infant's chest, and cried uncontrollably. I waited a minute or two. "Spend as much time with him as you want. The nurses are right outside the door and will check in occasionally. Let them know if you have any more questions."

I slowly left the room; and walked past the somber staff at the workstation. "I need a moment." Entering an empty room, I knelt by the bed and wept.

Teamwork

Mrs. Smith was an 87-year-old woman who lived alone and had a long history of hypertension and CHF. When her daughter went to visit that morning, she found her mother extremely short of breath and called 911. The paramedics established an IV line and gave her oxygen enroute to our ER. Upon initial exam she was anxious, markedly short of breath, hypoxic, and hypertensive. She had no chest pain. Her ECG was negative for acute ischemia. Physical examination revealed a bit of pink frothy sputum with coughing, JVD (distended jugular / neck veins), rales about 3/4 way up the posterior chest, and moderate edema of both lower legs. This was "Flash" pulmonary edema, a rapid accumulation of fluid in the lungs from heart failure.

This was a true medical emergency and could cause a cardiac arrest in minutes if not reversed. We administered 100 % oxygen by mask, gave a double dose of SL (sublingual / under the tongue) NTG (nitroglycerin, a blood vessel dilator), 5 mg of morphine (to decrease anxiety and blood pressure) IV push, and 40 mg of furosemide (a diuretic) IV push. We prepped for intubation, and obtained a portable chest X-ray (revealing moderate pulmonary edema). The nurses placed a foley catheter into the bladder to monitor urine output.

We watched at the bedside for about 10 minutes. Flash pulmonary edema was common. Patients would typically either worsen and require intubation, or "Turn the corner" and rapidly improve. This elderly woman rapidly improved. The oxygen level increased, and the RR, HR and BP all decreased beautifully. The foley catheter started flowing briskly with clear amber urine. The cough with frothy sputum disappeared. She was out of danger, but would require hospital admission for close monitoring, and to fine tune her medications to avoid a repeat episode.

We were a free-standing ER at that time. I called the hospital where her physicians were on staff and planned for transfer. The receiving ER physician advised using their helicopter transfer team. I indicated that the patient had arrived seriously ill, but improved markedly, and was stable for a routine ground transport (about 30 minutes by EMS). He wanted the patient transferred by the quickest route. Thinking it was unnecessary and too costly, I said, "The helicopter transfer might save 5 or 10 minutes, and the patient is now stable." He was insistent about using their air transport team. The final decision was up to the receiving hospital, so I reluctantly agreed.

About 20 minutes later the helicopter landed and their transfer team arrived. They were typically well trained and experienced, handling numerous transfers of critically ill patients from all over lower Michigan. The flight medical team (a PA and an RN) received a report from our nurses. I was close by, listening. After examining the patient, they planned intubation in the ER, to protect her airway and prevent having to perform a potentially difficult procedure while in flight.

I indicated that probably wasn't needed. The patient had continued to improve, her VS remained stable, and there was over 1,000 cc's (a liter) of urine in the foley bag. The chance of fluid reaccumulating in the lungs was very low. The two crew members said they were following flight transfer protocol and reviewed the case with the supervising base physician. Intubation was occasionally risky, but in this case it should be straightforward. Flight crews had extensive training and experience with airway management. The final decision was the responsibility of the transfer team. So I said, "Go ahead."

The ER was busy. I went to care for other patients. About 20 minutes later I poked my head back into their room. A disaster was in process. Both providers were anxious and sweating. They had just finished an attempt at intubation. The patient was unresponsive and paralyzed. There was blood around the patient's nose, mouth, and down her neck onto the bed. Worse yet were the VS were critical: the pulse ox was only 86% (significant hypoxia), and the HR 136. "Want me to help?" I asked.

"Yes, if you'd like," was their reply.

I called out to our staff, "We need the code team." Diane, RT arrived in seconds. She was talented and experienced. We ventilated the patient by BVM with 100 % oxygen and ensured a good fit with the mask and set out intubation equipment. The pulse ox monitor rose quickly to the high 90's. I ordered a dose of succinylcholine and attempted intubation. Inserting the laryngoscope, I couldn't visualize the vocal cords due to bright red blood bleeding in the posterior oral cavity. Diane had prepared two high volume suction catheters; we both suctioned the pharynx. Immediately the vocal cords appeared. As I inserted the ET (endotracheal / breathing tube), Diane put a gloved finger in the corner of the patient's mouth and pulled slightly, giving me an excellent view of the tube passing through the cords and into the trachea. I firmly held the ET tube and removed the stylet. Diane inflated the cuff to seal the airway and started ventilating. The in-line CO_2 (carbon dioxide) detector changed colors from yellow to purple, confirming placement into the trachea. CO_2 would only come from the lungs. The patient's oxygenation remained excellent, and the heart rate gradually diminished to normal. A portable chest X-ray confirmed good placement of the ET tube.

Mrs. Smith was stable again, out of danger. The flight crew members were taking notes and packing their equipment. They said nothing. Shortly thereafter, they whisked the patient out the EMS entrance to the helicopter for transfer to the inpatient hospital.

About two weeks later we received a short letter from the director of the air transport team about Mrs. Smith. She had done well and was discharged after a 6-day hospital stay. The last line was, "We would like to thank you for your offer of assistance." That was putting it mildly. My, "Offer of assistance," had saved the patient's life, and bailed the transfer team out.

I wrote back. I wasn't sure why the transfer team was hesitant to ask for assistance. It was readily available just outside the curtain of the resuscitation room. With bleeding in the posterior pharynx obscuring the vocal cords (from the transport team's initial attempts) the intubation procedure became extremely challenging. We were fortunate that our RT Diane was present. I indicated that as a young physician I had a similar experience that could have resulted in disaster. I recommended not hesitating, to ask for help early. They didn't reply.

―――――――――――

Epilepsy is a relatively common condition affecting about one percent of the population. It is a neurologic seizure disorder marked by recurrent episodes of sudden loss of consciousness and / or convulsions due to abnormal electrical activity in the brain. People not familiar with epilepsy are often terrified when observing a seizure. Suddenly someone drops to the ground unresponsive. Often the patient's eyes roll back. There can be jerking of the arms and legs, incontinence of urine, and gurgling, foaming saliva type respirations. This is followed by extreme sleepiness and then gradual awakening. The spell typically lasts a few minutes. However frightening seizures appear, they are usually not harmful to the patient (unless they are driving, bathing, swimming, etc).

Most patients with epilepsy have their seizures well controlled by medication, and live normal lives. A prolonged seizure (longer than five minutes), or one that keeps recurring without the patient returning to a normal level of consciousness is termed "Status epilepticus". Status epilepticus is rare but can occur in both adults and children. Most people with epilepsy will never have it. This is fortunate as status epilepticus can cause severe brain damage and death. After 30 to 60 minutes of continuous seizure activity significant damage to the patient is likely to begin. Status epilepticus is treatable, but often extremely challenging. Antiseizure medications can stop the episode, but the longer the seizure continues the less likely medications will work.

Our ER saw numerous pediatric patients. We were located in a growing community with a good school system and many young families. Most children brought to the ER are quite healthy and have relatively minor conditions: cuts, bruises, fractures, and infections. These are easily cared for and seldom require hospital admission. About one in a hundred pediatric patients required hospitalization. We'd call the attending pediatrician, discuss the case, and transfer the child by EMS or by car with the parents to the nearby pediatric hospital. Most of the pediatricians were extremely thankful during these (often late night) calls. Before the specialty of emergency medicine, pediatricians would handle all of these situations by phone or come into the hospital to see the child themselves.

After I'd been practicing in the ER for 10 years the nearby pediatric group hired Dr. Wells. He'd recently finished residency training. Dr. Wells was diligent, enthusiastic, and loved to talk. The downside was no matter how carefully we evaluated his patients when we called him about an admission, he would give us a thorough cross examination. He always wanted additional tests ordered and medications administered. These recommendations were typically performed after admission and were not necessary in the ER. We already started necessary treatment and stabilized the child. Dr. Wells would persist, often not "Accepting" the admission until we had followed his requests. This resulted in prolonged ER stays for his patients, delaying the hospital admission, and worsening our often-crowded department.

I was the physician director of the ER. So, after my partners and I had been "Interrogated" by young Dr. Wells many times I scheduled a meeting with him. I asked him about any concerns he had about the ability of our physicians to care for his patients. I indicated the ER was not set up for long periods of observation and treatment and discussed our goal to work as an efficient team in providing world class health care to his pediatric patients. During this meeting he was pleasant, responsive, and thankful for our efforts. However, this discussion had no effect on his behavior.

Phone calls to Dr. Wells still resulted in harassing questions and numerous additional requests.

Then one morning a mother rushed to the ER with her seizing daughter, Dorothy. Just as they arrived Dr. Wells was entering the hospital to round on his admitted pediatric patients. "Dr. Wells, can you help," she pleaded. All three were brought immediately to Room 1, Resuscitation by the triage nurse. I entered the room and recognized the seizing child.

She was one of four young children in the area that had epilepsy with frequent episodes of life-threatening status epilepticus. Many times, our routine antiseizure medications weren't effective, necessitating paralysis and intubation. All these patients had numerous medical problems and developmental delays. Most were on multiple antiseizure medications, which were changed frequently, and still not effective. These patients' presentations were common enough to our ER that we'd had special meetings about them. The latest guidelines for managing pediatric status epilepticus were posted in the resuscitation room. We added suggestions for using atypical or unusual antiseizure medications. These children were extremely challenging to care for. With their small size and active body jerking even routine procedures were difficult. Regular IV line placement was nearly impossible. After numerous ER visits most of their superficial veins were scarred and obliterated.

I went to the bedside and briefly examined the seizing child. Two nurses were attempting IV line placement. A respiratory therapist had arrived and was suctioning oral secretions and providing high flow oxygen by mask. The PALS crash cart was next to us. "Open the IO drill," I asked the tech. According to the mother, this seizure had started 25 minutes ago. At home she'd given rectal diazepam (an anti-seizure medication) as instructed. It didn't work. "We need to start a secure IV, either in the neck or interosseous in the leg, and perhaps intubate your daughter shortly," I advised.

"Are you a pediatrician?" the mother asked.

"No, Emergency Medicine."

She turned to Dr. Wells, "Will you take care of Dorothy?"

A long four or five seconds passed. Dr. Wells looked at the seizing child. It was likely a couple years since he last placed any IV line, maybe never drilling into the tibia for an IO line. His last intubation was probably many years before, the same for running a resuscitation for status epilepticus. He looked towards me, "Dr. Thomson, why don't you start."

"No problem." I grabbed the IO drill, fastened the pediatric tip, splashed betadine over the proximal tibia and drilled from slightly medial. After feeling a small "give" I removed the drill and jiggled the needle. It was stuck rigidly into the bone. I removed the stylet and flushed the needle with two cc's saline. Excellent flow. Beautiful. We had central IV access for medications. I watched the two RNs double checking the medication doses. "Push the Ativan, start the Dilantin drip, and get Phenobarbital ready. We'll follow the protocol," I instructed. A few minutes passed. The seizing continued. "Let's prep for RSI (rapid sequence intubation)." I moved to the head of the bed. The RT had already set out the airway equipment. We drew up sedative and paralytic medications, double checking the doses. I checked the laryngoscope light, blade, and ET tube size.

Pausing briefly, I looked over to the mother and Dr. Wells (both standing quietly past the foot of the bed), wondering if he wanted to do the intubation. The mother turned and looked at Dr. Wells. He was frozen solid, his feet glued to the floor. "I'll do the intubation," I said to no one in particular. The RSI went smoothly. I saw the vocal cords on the first attempt and passed the ET tube without difficulty. We secured the tube with tape. We reviewed the ventilator (breathing machine) settings and administered a long-acting paralytic. The patient's tonic clonic jerking extremities stopped. Most of the immediate danger had passed. We still needed to send Dorothy quickly to the pediatric ICU for brain wave monitoring, to ensure the electrical seizure activity in the brain had stopped.

I went to my workstation to place admitting orders and call the pediatric ICU doctor. A short time later the transfer team passed by, taking the child, monitors, medications, and ventilator down the hall to the elevator. The mother was with them. Dr. Wells stopped by my desk, hesitating.

"I'm just finishing the orders," I said.

"Uh, thank you Mark. I really appreciate it," said Dr. Wells.

"You're welcome," I replied. "Let's hope the child does well." After this episode we still had admissions and telephone discussions with Dr. Wells. The "Cross examinations" disappeared.

Compassion

Natalie, a young mother, raced Audrey, her 4-year-old daughter to triage. "She smashed her finger in the drawer." The child was anxious and distraught (like her mother). Audrey was tearful and crying vigorously. There was a large dish towel wrapped around the hand. We had the young child look away and carefully removed the towel. There was an ugly, swollen, and bloody fingertip. The nail was nearly avulsed (torn off) and some of the distal phalanx (bone) exposed.

This finger injury is very common in pediatric and adult patients. Any digit that gets slammed in a door, cupboard or drawer near the tip often has a similar pattern. The nail base gets ripped out of the paronychium (nail fold), the nail bed gets lacerated, and the bone that is just underneath becomes exposed. There can be a fair amount of bleeding and swelling. It does look gruesome, and (because of the sensitive innervation at the fingertip) is extremely painful.

The repair (especially after being performed a few times) is not tremendously difficult but does require careful attention to detail. It takes about 30 minutes. After a digital block (injection of a long-acting anesthetic) at the base of the finger, the wound is washed and irrigated thoroughly. Using good illumination, a rubber band tourniquet is applied at the base of the digit to control bleeding and allow for excellent visualization. The wound is inspected, checking for foreign material. Loss of bone is unusual. The nail bed laceration is re-approximated using absorbable sutures. The nail is placed back into its normal position in the paronychial fold and then sutured into place. The prognosis for complete healing and normal function is excellent.

I turned to the mother and said, "This is no problem. I can fix Audrey up and have you on your way shortly."

The mother was aghast, crossed her arms in front of her chest, and stared at me as if I was a cold and callous human being. Here she was with her daughter who almost lost part of her finger. "What do you mean? I saw a bone in there!" she said indignantly.

This was the second time I received a reaction like this. Now, I was beginning to understand. I was trying to be calm and reassuring, but somehow came across as uncaring. My approach certainly wasn't effective. What was routine and straightforward to me was a frightening emergency for the parents of young children. A more empathetic response was needed.

"Oh, you're correct. This is a significant injury to the fingertip. It certainly looks bad, because of all the blood and swelling, and there is bone exposed. The good news is we can carefully repair everything, save the bone and all of the tissue. She may lose the nail, but a new one will grow back in about 6 months. The prognosis is excellent. I have seen this type of injury many times and can carefully repair Audrey's fingertip. Your daughter's finger should be fine."

I repaired the injured finger in 25 minutes. There were no complications. Audrey tolerated the procedure well. Natalie settled down and was much happier. I should know, she's, my daughter.

Lynnette was in serious trouble. She was 23-years-old and dying from septic shock. She had been in good health with no history of medical problems. After missing her menstrual period, she went to an unlicensed clinic. Her pregnancy test was positive. Four days prior to this ER visit she returned to the same clinic and underwent an elective abortion. After the procedure she had a bit of spotting and mild abdominal pain. Yesterday evening she developed increased pain, a high fever, nausea and vomiting. Her roommate brought her in after finding her confused, weak and unable to stand this morning. The roommate was able to provide an accurate history.

Lynnette was weak, pale, and unable to answer questions. Her skin was cool, pale, and clammy. Her temperature was 103, respirations shallow and fast at 24, HR 172, and BP 60 / 40. We took her directly to resuscitation. The ER team placed her in a gown, applied a heart rate monitor, started oxygen, inserted two large bore IVs, and began a bolus of LR (lactated ringers). Simultaneously I performed a thorough exam. Significant findings included decreased LOC (level of consciousness), only grimacing to a sternal rub. Bimanual pelvic exam revealed diffuse uterine tenderness (moaning) and a foul smelling, dark vaginal discharge.

Her diagnosis was septic endometritis, a life-threatening uterine infection. Fortunately, it was rare. It was more common years before when elective abortions were illegal. This led to frequent "Backroom" abortions with unsterile equipment (or coat hangers). When these are used to scrape the interior lining of the uterus many serious infections occur, and occasionally result in the death of a healthy young woman. This was the first case I had seen since medical school.

I returned to the workstation to enter orders just as Evelyn (a full time RN) arrived with numerous vials of blood. "Check her BP every few minutes and let me know if it doesn't come up. We may have to start norepinephrine (a vasoconstricting medicine to increase BP). I'm worried if this young woman doesn't respond to fluids her mortality risk is extremely high."

Evelyn replied, "Serves her right." I glanced up, unsure if I'd heard her correctly. Evelyn was looking directly at me. She meant for me to hear it. Shocked at the comment, I said nothing.

I paged the intensivist and reviewed the antibiotic choice. We started clindamycin and gentamicin. Fortunately, the blood pressure and heart rate improved, and Lynnette became alert. I added two more liters of IV fluid to her orders. She was transferred in critical but stable condition to the ICU. She survived and was discharged five days later. The IV fluids and antibiotics saved her life.

This episode troubled me for quite some time. I had witnessed Evelyn being empathetic in the past but was surprised in this instance with her lack of compassion. Our ER was run by a Catholic hospital which didn't provide abortions. I knew Evelyn was a dedicated church going Catholic, and assumed she was against elective abortions. However, we knew nothing about the patient's past, her family and social life, and no details about the pregnancy or current living situation.

Nearly all women are hesitant when giving their medical history of an elective abortion, obvious they come to that decision after serious consideration. I wanted to practice medicine with human understanding, and integrity. Who was I to judge? There is no way to learn all the facts regarding these situations. I decided to leave blame, guilt and punishment for another time and place.

———————————

A 46-year-old woman presented to the ER with abdominal pain. She had been in excellent health. This was her first visit to an emergency department. She didn't even have a family doctor. She stopped getting pap smears after menopause. She was nulliparous (had not borne offspring). Over the past month she noted some mild diffuse abdominal discomfort and felt bloated. She had gained a few pounds and noticed her clothes were tight around her waist. The rest of her medical history was unremarkable. On general appearance she was calm but concerned. The complete physical examination was negative. The abdomen was nontender, without palpable masses or any fluid wave. I couldn't find any abnormality. Her pelvic exam was negative.

"I'm not sure the cause of your symptoms. We can send off some routine laboratory studies and get an abdominal and pelvic ultrasound." She easily agreed, wanting investigation of her symptoms.

The lab tests were normal. Jeannie, the US technician, brought the patient back to the ER, and looked seriously concerned. She said, "The radiologist will call you with the US report."

Shortly, I received the call. "Mark, this is bad news. I see a pelvic mass, a small amount of free fluid in the abdomen, and numerous small lesions on the peritoneum lining (interior abdominal wall). This is peritoneal carcinomatosis, likely from ovarian cancer, stage

III or IV." While listening I had brought up the films on the computer, reviewing the images myself.

"How sure are you?" I asked.

"Almost 100 percent. I can't believe anything else can look like this. Of course, you need a biopsy for confirmation."

I called our gynecologic oncologist. He could see the patient in his office the next evening.

It is difficult to decide how much information to give patients about a diagnosis like this. With such a serious illness it doesn't seem right to tell them they have a spot or a lump that needs further evaluation. The patient waits anxiously to see their doctor or oncologist, then are told they have advanced metastatic cancer. I didn't want to give false hope. On the other hand, I didn't want to tell of an extremely poor prognosis and take hope away. Whenever possible, it is best to leave room for hope. Of course, you would hate to say the patient has cancer and then the biopsy returns negative. That would be extremely unlikely in this case. There are usually many questions about prognosis, best answered by an oncologist. In her case I knew the prognosis. It was horrible, most patients dying within six to nine months.

I pulled her chart and reviewed it again. She was single and had come to the ER by herself. Beth, her nurse, was sitting next to me and heard my discussions with radiology and oncology. "What are you going to tell her?" she asked.

"I'm not sure," I said and walked slowly to the patient's room. "I've got your test results. Are there any friends or family members nearby?" I sat down. She quietly shook her head no, sensing what was coming. I spoke deliberately, "Your lab tests are normal, but there were abnormalities on the ultrasound. I reviewed the scan with the radiologist. There is a mass in your pelvis, and numerous lesions on the abdominal wall. It's likely ovarian cancer." I waited for a response.

She said, "I thought so. I read on the internet about weight gain and bloating. Are those lesions the cancer spreading?"

"Most likely," I replied. She must have read about the horrible prognosis of metastatic ovarian cancer. There was a short silence. I was not prepared for her response.

"I'll bet this isn't easy for you, breaking bad news to patients."

I had just confirmed her suspicions and given her a virtual death sentence. Now, her thoughts were about me. Incredible. I had to think for a moment. "You're right about that; it's always difficult. Thank you." I reviewed her discharge instructions with her. She would be able to see the oncologist. I went back to the workstation.

Beth asked, "How did she take it? What did she say?"

"I can hardly believe it. I told her it was metastatic ovarian cancer. She knows she's in serious trouble. After I told her the diagnosis the only thing she asked was how I was doing." We sat in silence, struggling to hold back tears.

Sore Throat

I started an evening shift and picked up the first chart in the rack. The chief complaint was: 10-year-old boy with a sore throat. This was usually a quick encounter. Viral pharyngitis or a bacterial "Strep throat" infection were common ER diagnoses in the winter months. I entered the patient's room and started taking the history. Immediately I realized this would not be a simple brief visit. The nurses had put the child into a gown. He was laying down on the bed, not just sitting on the edge. Both parents had come with him to the ER and were on chairs near the head of the bead. The father answered my questions.

Looking over the youngster was troubling. He was pale, had quick shallow breaths and looked frightened. The vital signs were moderately abnormal: 101.6 temp; RR: 24 (12-20 is normal) HR 118 (60-100). "He's been sick now for two weeks. First, we took him to an UC (Urgent Care). They diagnosed a viral URI (upper respiratory infection / cold). A few days later we saw our family doctor. The strep test was negative. He gradually got worse, so we went back three days ago and were given a Rx for an antibiotic. He's no better, in fact he is getting worse. His fever and sore throat are worse, he has no appetite, he's weak and lethargic. We don't want to leave until we get to the bottom of this." Both parents were calm, but also were firm and serious. They maintained eye contact throughout the patient history.

I'd been standing at the foot of the bed listening and observing the child. He wasn't just a bit pale, but ghostly white. I could see his abdomen was distended through the thin hospital gown. Most concerning was the rash on his legs. Multiple tiny, dark purplish spots were visible, more numerous the lower down towards the ankles and feet. The spots didn't blanch (lighten in color under finger pressure). This was a dreadful petechial rash, often found with critical infections and disease. I'd only seen this a half dozen times; the outcome frequently bad.

"You won't be taking him home tonight. Your son is seriously ill and needs to be admitted. We'll find out the cause." It was the most direct I'd ever spoken to parents. I hadn't even finished my physical exam or gotten any test results. It was obvious, this child was in danger. I examined him head to toe. No photophobia and his neck was supple (no meningitis) and lung auscultation clear (no pneumonia). His heart rate was fast, but pulses were strong. No septic shock. Palpating the abdomen, I found a markedly enlarged liver and spleen. Tapping gently confirmed a fluid wave, indicating abnormal fluid in the abdominal cavity. There were nontender, enlarged lymph nodes in his neck and groin. I ordered a full panel of blood and urine tests. An IV was started and a fluid bolus given. The chest X-ray was negative.

About 30 minutes later Lynn, the laboratory technician, called and asked that I come over to review the blood smear. This was unusual. I would rarely check microscope slides, except for meningitis.

"What's up?" I asked.

"His WBC count is massively elevated, and look," she motioned to the microscope.

At first, I was puzzled. There were some pale RBCs (Red Blood Cells) but numerous obviously abnormal WBC's. They all had large, irregular, black densities in the nuclei. I hadn't seen a slide

111

like this since Histology class in medical school. "This looks like some horrible leukemia," I said.

"Yes," Lynn replied.

I didn't want to believe it, "Are you absolutely sure? Not a strange virus or Mononucleosis?"

"I'm sure. I've been preparing blood and bone marrow slides for Hem / Onc (hematology and oncology) for years."

I suddenly felt heavy on the stool. It took an effort to stand. I had to inform the parents.

"The initial tests have returned. I reviewed the slides in the lab. It's very likely your son has leukemia." I waited for the bad news to sink in. Reactions to suddenly hearing bad news is extremely variable. Denial, anger, tears. Sometimes all three.

These parents remained quiet and calm, "What's the next step?" They seemed relieved in some way. They must have suspected something was seriously wrong. I had confirmed their fears. They were resolute, ready to do whatever was necessary for their son. It was one of the most impressive moments I'd ever witnessed.

Trying to be optimistic, I mentioned that a number of childhood leukemias do respond to treatment. Their son would be transferred to the nearby pediatric hospital. Hem / Onc would be consulted, and many additional tests performed. Likely a bone marrow biopsy. We would start IV antibiotics, because of his fever a serious infection could be present. I rechecked his VS, they were improving. He was transferred in stable condition, his future uncertain.

Chief complaint, "Trouble swallowing." In the ENT room was a 35-year-old woman, "It started a few weeks ago. First it was intermittent, but gradually got worse. My throat is sore, it feels like a tightness or a lump or something is stuck." She was now having trouble eating solid food, liquids were okay, and she had very little appetite. No fever or pain, no sinus congestion or drainage, no cough or hoarseness, no nausea or vomiting, no reflux or heartburn. She never had anything like this in the past. Her past medical history was negative. There was no history of allergies. She was a nonsmoker, wasn't on any medications, and didn't think she could be pregnant.

Her exam didn't reveal any pathology. Careful palpation of her neck revealed a few small, nontender cervical lymph nodes (a normal finding). There was no tenderness, and a normal thyroid gland. She was well hydrated with moist mucous membranes, there was no hoarseness. I was stumped. Certainly, this wasn't likely anything serious. I sent off a strep screen and CBC. A minor work up, it would give me a chance to think.

The test results returned shortly. All were normal. When the history and physical exam are negative, dysphagia (trouble swallowing) is commonly due to stress and anxiety. An old term was globus hystericus. She certainly didn't appear anxious or hypochondriacal. In fact, she was somewhat somber, with a mildly flat affect. I returned to the ENT room. Taking just a minute, I used our flexible ENT scope (fiber optic nasopharyngeal laryngoscope) to inspect her posterior pharynx and vocal cords. No foreign body, perfectly normal. I assured her I didn't find anything serious. One possibility was occult esophageal reflux. "Try some antacids every night before bedtime. If your symptoms don't entirely resolve over the next week, then call the ENT specialist on your discharge instructions. The nurse will bring your paperwork."

A short time later her nurse approached me. "Dr. Thomson, you know the lady in the ENT room? She wants to talk to you."

"What about?" I replied.

"It's about her son. Do you remember the young boy we saw about 6 months ago with leukemia?"

I absolutely did and would never forget it. I had also seen something on the TV news about him. It was a story of a young boy with leukemia that needed a bone marrow transplant. They were having trouble finding a match. They encouraged everyone to donate blood and become registered as a bone marrow donor. That wasn't good news. It meant his chemotherapy wasn't effective. Why did she want to talk to me? I recalled being direct with her and her husband about the young boy's critical illness. Was I too harsh? Was she upset that I was so blunt? Had I made some mistake?

I walked back to the ENT room to face her. "Do you remember treating my son a few months ago," she asked.

"Yes. I didn't recognize you, but the nurses told me who you were."

"Well," she said, "I just wanted to thank you." I thought, what did I do? I had told them their son had a critical and life-threatening illness. "The doctors we saw (before you) told us it wasn't anything serious, just a virus or throat infection. You knew right away." By the time I saw him, the horrible petechial rash had appeared.

"What happened after he was admitted?" I asked. "They started chemotherapy. At first it seemed to work, but then he relapsed. We tried to find a match for a bone marrow transplant but couldn't. He died one month ago."

My eyes filled with tears. Jaw trembling, I tried to respond but couldn't speak. I bowed my head and took her hand. I tried again but still couldn't speak. We spent some time in silence. I lifted my eyes to catch her gaze and nodded. I turned slowly, left the room, walked down the hall, and wept.

Stoic Patients

On a Saturday afternoon in August a 43-year-old man presented with chest pain. "Hello, I'm Dr. Thomson, tell me about your chest pain." He related that he was working underneath his truck changing the water pump. His arms were above him when he noticed some mild discomfort in his chest, and his arms felt heavy. He pushed himself out from under the truck. After about 5 or 10 minutes he felt better. He started to work again, using some big wrenches, and the same thing happened. He stopped and rested again; the discomfort went away. Because it happened twice, and he was a smoker, he wanted to get it checked out. There was no shortness of breath, nausea, or vomiting. He denied any other symptoms. I asked him if there was any sweating during the episodes. He said he'd been sweating before and after due to the muggy, hot day, about 88 degrees. His history was otherwise unremarkable. Past medical and family histories were negative. No heart disease, no medical problems. He seemed stoic. This was his first time in an ER. His exam was normal. He was asymptomatic. No tenderness of his arms, shoulder, or chest wall. The ECG was perfect. "We'll get some routine lab tests, some cardiac enzymes, and a chest X-ray.

After about an hour the lab tests returned. Everything was normal, including the troponin (heart enzyme test). The chest X-ray was negative. I calculated his HEART SCORE (History, ECG, Age, Risk Factors, Troponin / cardiac enzyme scoring system). It was 3 out of 10. This meant his risk of a heart attack was low. Under two percent within the next month. I returned to the patient's room and discussed his results. "Your test results are normal. I can't find anything serious. The chest discomfort and arm heaviness could be due to working under your truck on such a hot day. However, you're over 40 and a smoker so it's important for you to follow up with your doctor in the next few days. Of course, you should quit smoking."

He reached into his shirt pocket, grabbed a pack of cigarettes, and threw them in the trash. "No problem, I'm done with these." he said dramatically. He seemed relieved.

The next day I arrived just before 7 AM to begin my shift. Dr. Mark Rosenwasser the overnight physician said, "Let's sign out in the back." I knew something was up as we left the workstation. The nurses were quiet and watching intently as we walked to the office.

Mark asked, "Do you remember the 43-year-old with chest pain you saw yesterday?"

I nodded, "Yes." A conversation starting like this was usually delivering bad news.

"Well, EMS brought him back about 11 PM in full arrest. His wife found him unresponsive in bed. He was flatline, we couldn't revive him."

I sat in stunned silence, not wanting to believe what I had just been told. My mouth was dry, my heart pounding. "Are you sure it was the same patient?" praying there had been a mistake.

"Yes. I checked the medical record, everything was negative. I'd have sent him home too," he said, trying to console me. I barely heard him.

"Think it was a heart attack, an arrhythmia?" I asked.

"Most likely. Probably not a PE (pulmonary embolism) or aortic dissection. The ME (Medical Examiner) is doing a post (autopsy)." The autopsy would show a 95 % blockage in the LAD (left anterior descending), the largest artery supplying blood to the heart. "I know you've got the shift to work today. Take your time. I have a few patients to dispo and will be in the department for a while. I thought it best for me to fill you in."

I stumbled my way through the day. The nurses were quiet and subdued. They left me alone. My mind was racing. Every spare moment I went back to inspect his medical record. Even with a microscopic hindsight review I couldn't find anything else. He was at low risk. I pulled up the literature on the "HEART SCORE" which I already knew well. Chest pain was such a frequent complaint I used the scoring system almost daily. Our department followed those guidelines. Recommendations for low-risk patients were to discharge for close outpatient follow up. That didn't make me feel any better. My patient was dead.

I could hardly sleep over the next few weeks. The case went through our Quality Assurance Review, routine for these occurrences. The conclusion was the HEART SCORE was 3. You followed the guidelines. They couldn't find any mistakes. During the discussions many of the senior physicians admitted to sending a patient home that soon returned with a heart attack. I felt a minuscule better but still couldn't sleep. I kept thinking about his wife, finding him down. I didn't know if they had children. I hadn't asked. It wasn't in his chart.

The case would haunt me. It affected my clinical practice. I resented every patient that complained of chest pain. I'd perform a complete cardiac work up on every one of them, even if they had another obvious diagnosis. At a minimum, I would hold patients in the ER for four hours and repeat the troponin (cardiac enzyme). Like most ER doctors I would see about 100 patients a year with chest pain. If a low-risk patient was about two percent chance of heart attack over the next month, that would be one or two patients a year. I didn't want another patient with a bad outcome. I sent many patients to the observation unit for cardiac consultation and possible stress testing. I was overly cautious. It took years for me to follow routine practice guidelines.

I entered room 11 and found a young woman, resting comfortably. She was 36-years-old and came to the ER complaining of a headache (HA). "Tell me the details about your headache."

She had returned home from grocery shopping and suddenly developed a HA on the left side. It was a sharp moderately severe pain, about "6 out of 10." It made her stop putting the groceries away and lay down for a while. She seldom had headaches in the past. When she did, they were temporal or generalized and more of a tension or band type pain. It was not the worst headache of her life. The pain didn't radiate. There was no fall or trauma, no nausea or vomiting, no syncope or seizure. The pain was a "1" now. "I almost didn't come in," she said. Her past medical history was unremarkable. She wasn't pregnant. Her exam was negative, she was not in any distress. Her neck was supple, the neurologic exam was normal.

The question was what work up should I do? We saw patients with a HA almost every shift. The vast majority have no serious illness. Most are migraine or tension headaches. The differential diagnosis however is long and includes many serious life-threatening conditions: subarachnoid hemorrhage, stroke, blood clots, meningitis, encephalitis, trauma, brain tumors, etc. Usually there are "Red Flags" found on the history or exam, which indicate a likely serious cause for the headache. These include: a thunderclap onset, 10 out of 10 pain, the worst HA of your life, fever, photophobia and stiff neck, seizure, syncope, a fall or trauma, pregnancy or recently postpartum, taking blood thinning medication, persistent nausea and vomiting, and any stroke type symptoms or signs on exam, double vision, facial weakness, slurred speech, and numbness or weakness in the arms or legs. I'm sure there are a few more. The only one this patient had was the sudden onset. She appeared comfortable, and the pain was only a 1 out of 10. It concerned me that she had to stop what she was doing. She seemed stoic, but the HA concerned her enough to come to the ER. I decided to perform the complete HA work up.

We drew blood for tests and obtained a CT scan of the head without contrast. The CT scan report returned in 30 minutes; it was perfectly normal. I reviewed it with the radiologist. I went back to see her. She was resting comfortably. Pain still rated a 1. "Your CT scan is normal. The only remaining concern I have is the possibility you could have a small, leaking aneurysm. The CT scan is about 98 % accurate at finding those. About 2 % can be missed. The danger from missing a leaking aneurysm is that it could rebleed in the next few days. That can cause a massive stroke, even death. I think the safest plan is to obtain spinal fluid by doing a spinal tap. We would check the fluid under a microscope for blood. If the fluid is clear, then the risk of an aneurysm is pretty much ruled out." It was my usual speech.

"Oh yes, go ahead," she readily agreed.

That surprised me. She was more concerned than she was letting on. I had been through similar discussions literally hundreds of times, and most patients were hesitant (thinking about having a spinal tap with a long needle poking into their lower back). I had performed about four hundred spinal taps. Lumbar punctures and evaluations for possible aneurysms or meningitis were common for me. Obviously not common for the patient.

I returned with the LP kit, and briefly described the procedure in more detail. A few minutes later I slowly advanced the 22 gauge (thin) spinal needle about 3 cm into the L3 - L4 interspace. When I felt a small give and a slight pop, I stopped advancing the needle. Upon removing the stylet, out dripped what looked like strawberry Kool-Aid. Normal spinal fluid is clear. This could only be blood. "There is some blood with your spinal fluid. There has to be some bleeding around your brain. You may have a small aneurysm. Your neurologic exam is normal, so your prognosis is pretty good. You will be admitted for more testing."

I sent the spinal fluid to the lab then walked directly back to the radiology reading room. Dr. James Sellis, an experienced radiologist, was reading CT scans that day. "Hey Jim, can you bring back up the CT scan on the woman in room 11? I just did an LP and there was obvious blood. She must have an aneurysm or subarachnoid hemorrhage." He pulled up the images. We reviewed them together.

"Even in hindsight, I can't find anything," he said.

I spoke with the NS (neurosurgeon). He said he was just finishing a case in the OR, he would see her shortly. She was admitted. Later that evening, the NS called back, "The cerebral angiogram was positive. She had an 8 mm aneurysm. We were able to coil it without any complications. I couldn't see anything on her head CT either. By doing the spinal tap you likely saved her life."

It felt good to hear that, but I was also spooked a bit. I had considered letting her go home without the HA work up. I remembered the stoic man with chest pain (I'd recently sent home) who died. That experience may have been the difference in deciding to order the CT and perform the LP.

Level One Trauma

It was a chaotic night. One of my partners had a medical emergency himself the day before, so I was working his shift at our hospital in Southfield, Michigan. It was located in an area with a fair amount of gun and knife activity. The ER and waiting rooms were full and then three trauma patients arrived simultaneously. Two gunshot victims and one patient with a knife wound to the head. There were three ER docs. Two of my partners saw the gunshot victims with the trauma team in the two trauma rooms. I was assigned the knife wound patient and one nurse aid as an assistant.

My patient Betty was a 24-year-old woman who admitted she was at a party and, "Had one beer". She insisted that she was, "Sitting on the porch, minding my own business," when completely out of the blue another woman came up from behind her and, "For no reason at all," pulled out a knife and stabbed her in the head.

This hardly seemed believable, but the absolute detailed truthful history wasn't important for my treatment. She also happened to know the two gunshot victims. All ERs are required to notify the local police when treating any patient who was a likely victim of interpersonal violence. The police were already in the ER. I would let them sort out the facts of the altercation.

Betty was minimally anxious and incredibly calm. Especially considering the blood squirting from her scalp wound whenever she let up pressure on the wound dressing. The right side of her head, face, neck, chest, and abdomen was saturated in blood. At times, a small amount of blood can appear impressively large. Likely in this case. The GCS (Glascow Coma Score) was 15 (no neurologic deficit). Her VS were normal, her skin color pink, and conjunctival membranes (around the eye) were not pale. She denied other injuries.

My assistant placed her in a gown. I did the primary trauma survey exam. It was normal. The secondary detailed exam revealed only the scalp wound. No other injuries. My assistant and I opened the suture repair kit, prepared a syringe with lidocaine and epinephrine (an anesthetic with a vasoconstrictor to slow any bleeding), donned gowns, gloves, face shields and aimed the overhead light towards the scalp wound. My assistant let up pressure on the wound dressing. I found a large scalp vessel squirting bright red pulsatile arterial blood. In a few seconds I injected the local anesthetic into nearby tissue and stopped the bleeding with pressure.

After three minutes we released pressure once again. There was minimal active bleeding. The wound was curved and 10 cm long (4 inches), there were no foreign bodies. Most importantly I had an excellent view. The skull was completely smooth and intact, by both visual inspection and palpation. There was no skull or brain injury. I placed one size 00 (large diameter, strong) silk suture around the scalp arterial bleeding site. Then closed the wound with 14 staples from the large staple gun in the trauma wound kit. (Staples from the small staple gun work poorly for deep scalp lacerations). Bacitracin ointment over the wound, a dT booster shot, and Betty in her hospital gown was ready for discharge. Her repeat GCS score and VS were perfectly normal. In a total of 25 minutes, she was ready to.

I prepared the discharge instructions as Wendy the charge nurse came by. "How's the patient with the knife wound doing?" she asked.

"Beautifully," I said. "Nothing but a large scalp laceration. I put about a dozen staples in. She is ready for discharge."

"That's impossible, with all that blood!" Wendy stated, incredulous.

"The bleeding has stopped. Her VS are normal," I explained.

"How was the CT scan?" Wendy demanded.

"I didn't do one. It wasn't needed," I said.

"How do you know the knife didn't go into the brain?"

"I was able to inspect the skull completely, smooth and intact," I answered.

She looked at me as if I was from another planet. I barely knew Wendy, having rarely taken shifts in the Southfield ER. "Have you worked in a trauma center?" she asked.

"No, just as the single physician in the Novi ER."

"I'm having the trauma team take a look at her," she said.

I thought about arguing with her, but knew I was the odd man out. My ER partners were swamped and had no time to sort this out. I put in the order for a trauma consultation. The trauma team saw Betty about an hour later. They ordered the complete trauma panel of blood tests, plain skull X-rays and a CT scan of the head with bone windows (to see the bone better). Another three hours passed. All the lab tests, X-rays and CT scans were normal, except the hemoglobin was slightly low at 12.6 (normal 13-15 in our lab). They cleared her for discharge. Wendy felt better. Betty was still being questioned by police. The patient's bill was likely quadrupled by the trauma consultation. I made a note to follow up and cancel the charges.

By 2000 our ER yearly patient census increased, and physician staffing now included double coverage from noon until midnight. One slow evening I was working with Dr. Richard Wagner. Rich loved to hunt and fish and was a good storyteller. His many adventures included trophy animals with large horns or antlers. I was certain he embellished the tales until one day he brought impressive pictures as proof. I had tried to keep up but had never shot a big buck, and most of my fish stories were about chasing nine-inch-long brook trout. He was regaling me about tracking a big bear through thick timber in a western Canadian province when the ER received an urgent EMS call, "We're enroute with a level one trauma patient, a young woman ejected from a rollover MVA (Motor Vehicle Accident), and has head, facial and chest injuries."

We asked, "Do you know you're calling Providence ER in Novi?" We were not a Level One Trauma Center. The EMS protocol was to bypass all ERs and take critical trauma patients directly to the level one center (where trauma surgeons and ORs were readily available, and patient outcomes improved). EMS replied, "Yes, but we cannot establish an airway. The patient won't make it. We're one minute out." Our charge nurse glanced at me for approval. I gave the thumbs up sign. She said, "Okay, we'll be ready." We ran to the resuscitation room and opened the trauma supply cupboards.

"Rich, I'll manage the airway. You do any other procedure," I said. Seconds later, the EMS entrance doors opened. The paramedics swept in with the young woman. She was minimally responsive (with an occasional groan), pale, hypoxic and tachycardic. The paramedics were trying to ventilate with a BVM but having difficulty. Bloody, foamy liquid was coming out from her mouth. The patient was likely aspirating. Her face had dirty abrasions, significant bruising and swelling, and active bleeding from the nose. They couldn't get a good fit with the face mask.

The patient was dying. She needed a secure airway immediately. There were three options, all extremely challenging. Oral endotracheal intubation, a Combitube blindly jammed down her throat into either the esophagus or trachea, or a surgical airway in her anterior neck. All had significant risks and complications. "I'll try oral intubation first," I called out to the team. Dr. Wagner listened to the chest and found markedly decreased breath sounds indicating a large pneumothorax (collapsed lung) on the right side. "She needs a chest tube," he said.

The paramedics had removed the front portion of the immobilizing cervical collar when trying to ventilate the patient. I asked one of them to provide in-line stabilization of the head and neck (to avoid worsening a potential cervical spine injury). Our RT briefly suctioned the oral cavity. I placed an oral airway (small plastic block to open the mouth and keep the tongue from occluding the pharynx). The RT bagged the patient with 100 percent oxygen while I held the mask tightly over the patient's nose and mouth. With a few puffs, the pulse ox reading (oxygenation) improved. I noticed the upper incisors (teeth) were intact, but the maxilla (upper jaw) was freely moveable. This was a Lefort fracture, the facial bones were broken away from the skull.

I attempted intubation using a curved blade laryngoscope. Following the tongue, I was able to glide the tip of the blade towards the vallecula (junction of the epiglottis and tongue). I lifted the scope but couldn't see the vocal cords. Even with suctioning, there was too much frothy blood. Then, a small miracle happened. I noted some active bubbling. The patient had exhaled. I recalled a tip about intubating children with epiglottitis and severe throat swelling. "Try to advance the ET tube through the bubbles." I gently pushed the tip of the ET tube through the middle of the foamy bubbles. There was no resistance. "I must be in the trachea!" We inflated the ET tube cuff with a small syringe, attached the bag with 100 % oxygen to the proximal end and ventilated the patient a few times. There was excellent color change in the inline CO_2 detector device confirming placement into the trachea. After suctioning the ET tube, the patient's oxygen reading raced up to normal. Her tachycardia improved. Her airway was now secure. We placed the cervical collar back into position.

I looked up as Rich was pushing a large chest tube with a trocar (a long, thin surgical instrument with a sharp three-sided tip enclosed in a tube) through an incision he'd made in the right axilla. There was an obvious pop as he broke through the pleura (inner lining of the chest wall) and into the chest cavity. He advanced the tube past the end of the trocar, then placed a couple of large sutures for stabilization. Hooking the chest tube to a "Pleur Evac" (chest drainage system) with suction, we observed a small amount of blood and a moderate amount of air being removed. Repeat chest auscultation revealed good breath sounds. The pneumothorax was resolved. There was no time for confirmatory X-rays.

We hadn't moved the patient from the EMS cart. The paramedics scurried back to the ambulance with the young woman and raced away to the trauma center. They'd been in our ER for about 10 minutes. In his trauma survey exam Dr. Wagner hadn't found any other life-threatening injuries. We hoped for the best. This case presented so quickly I hadn't felt nervous. In the immediate aftermath I noticed my heart pounding, apprehensive about her outcome.

About two months later the triage nurse came into the back of the ER and said, "Dr. Thomson, there is someone who wants to see you."

"Who is it? I asked, somewhat concerned."

"Don't worry. You'll want to see them," she said.

I walked to the waiting room. A young woman was standing next to her mother, "Are you Dr. Thomson?"

"Yes," I nodded in reply.

"Don't you recognize me?" she asked.

"Uh no, sorry, I don't,"

She smiled and started laughing, "Well, I don't recognize you either. You saved my life! I was a car accident patient. You put some tubes into me. The trauma center doctors said you saved my life."

"Oh, I remember you now. Our whole team saved your life. You look great!" I had been worried about possible brain damage. She sounded and appeared perfectly normal. She stepped forward and we shared a long embrace, both shedding tears of joy.

Live Better Electrically

"Live Better Electrically," is a slogan from the 1950s, encouraging home electrification. It applies well to certain cardiac emergencies. ER physicians spend most of their time performing histories and exams. There's charting, order entries, discussions, and consultations. Procedures are numerous. Common ones include intubation, central IV lines, joint and fracture reductions, and wound care. Less common would include electrical cardioversion and defibrillation, lumbar punctures, and thoracostomy (chest) tubes. Rare procedures: pericardiocentesis, intraosseous line insertion and lateral canthotomy.

I had been practicing in the ER for a few years. A 50-year-old woman was brought in by family members with mild substernal, "Heartburn." As I began taking her history, she became lightheaded. Looking at the HR monitor I could see a fast, regular, wide rhythm about 200 beats per minute, V Tach (Ventricular tachycardia). "We need 200 joules for cardioversion. Get the pads on her chest." Within seconds we were ready. The patient was still conscious. "Ok. Everybody clear. Go ahead, shock." The patient jerked and let out a loud moan from the electrical jolt. She converted to a normal rhythm with frequent short runs of VT. I reviewed the ECG. There was definite ST segment elevation in the inferior leads. She was having a myocardial infarction.

This was before giving patients thrombolytics or transferring patients to the cardiac cath lab to directly open the blocked arteries. She had multiple recurrent episodes of longer VT all responding to cardioversion. Every minute or so we had to shock her. Early on she remained conscious, moaning loudly with each shock. We followed ACLS (advanced cardiac life support) protocol and administered numerous antiarrhythmic medications including lidocaine, procainamide, and bretylium. After 15 to 20 shocks, she didn't regain consciousness, and I couldn't palpate any pulses. We began chest compressions and went to unsynchronized cardioversion. Our electric shocks would occasionally restore a normal sinus rhythm, but quickly degenerate. She went into Ventricular fib (fibrillation). I ordered additional medication: epinephrine and magnesium and increased the Joules (amount of electricity) to 360. I intubated her without difficulty. She was completely unconscious. Her arrhythmia persisted. Nothing worked. A feeling of hopelessness came over the room. Additional shocks. We kept going. I'd never had a patient survive after more than 10 to 12 shocks. We were out of options. There were no more medications to give. I was considering stopping the resuscitation. We were up to 50 shocks.

Suddenly, the normal sinus rhythm persisted. The V fib and V tach resolved. She even had pulses! Unbelievable. I have no idea why she finally stopped having the lethal arrhythmias. The medications had been on board for quite some time. Maybe a miracle. She was admitted and transferred to the CCU. The whole episode lasted nearly one hour. I thought she would have significant heart or brain damage. I followed up with the cardiologist about a week later. He told me she was discharged from the hospital in good condition, including her neurologic function! Was it the same patient? I made him repeat it. "Yes, yes. She's doing well." To this day I can hardly believe it.

A couple of years later a 63-year-old man with a history of syncope drove himself to the ER. He denied chest pain or any other symptoms. "I was standing in the kitchen, then suddenly felt lightheaded. I broke into a sweat, then woke up on the floor." He denied headache, neck pain, abdominal pain, nausea, vomiting, diarrhea, bleeding, or incontinence. His past medical history was unremarkable, no seizures, no cardiac problems. His exam was negative. The ECG normal.

The staff placed him on a cardiac monitor and started an IV. I went to the workstation and ordered routine labs. A nurse called, "Dr. Thomson, come quick!! He's in V fib.

Checking, the patient was unconscious, unresponsive, pale, and diaphoretic. No pulses, the monitor showed V fib. I ordered 360 Joules for defibrillation. It worked, NSR (Normal Sinus Rhythm) restored. But only for a moment. The patient had stirred and moaned weakly. Less than a minute passed before more V fib. We shocked him again. Just like before, NSR was restored. We were able to obtain another ECG in between episodes of V fib. There was no ischemia (heart attack). He went back into V fib numerous times and was defibrillated each time.

We began CPR. I intubated the patient. Following ACLS guidelines, multiple rounds of medications were given, additional defibrillations. Each time returning the patient to NSR briefly. The lab studies returned, all, normal. Up to 30 shocks, 40. Now fine (low voltage) V fib. Continued CPR, more shocks, at least 50. Asystole developed on the heart monitor, complete flat line. I tried a pacemaker (inserting a wire through the neck down into the heart). No capture, no heartbeat. I called the code (stopping the resuscitation) and pronounced the patient dead.

The room was silent. We see a lot of death and dying in the ER. Most occurring in patients near the end of life or presenting with critical signs and symptoms in progress. To have someone enter the department walking, talking, looking healthy and then crash and not be resuscitated was uncommon. Processing what happened is difficult. What was the cause? Why did interventions (that normally work) fail? Could we have done anything differently? Those are unanswered questions from families and ER staff alike. The younger the patient, the more traumatic it is. These cases stay in your memory for years. Most of the time answers do not appear.

That same day, about an hour later, a pregnant woman rushed into the ER through our front entrance. "The baby's coming," she said urgently. The staff walked with her to the nearest empty room. She was obviously pregnant and near term, (with a large protruding abdomen). In a moment she was placed in a gown. "I have to push," she hollered.

I lifted the gown. The baby's head was crowning (showing at the vaginal opening). "Go ahead," I answered. She took a deep breath, held it, and with one heroic push the infant's head emerged. "One more push, a little one," I instructed. Out slid the newborn, a baby girl. I placed the infant on the mother's chest. The delivery had taken about two minutes.

The obstetrician arrived; she'd been finishing a cesarean section upstairs. I was beginning to suture a small tear in the perineum, the OB observing over my shoulder. "Want to do the repair? I asked.

"You're doing fine Mark, keep going," she answered. She double checked the mother. I did the newborn exam. Finishing by counting the fingers and toes. The baby's APGAR scores were 8 and 9, everything was normal. The infant's skin was pink, and warm, she had already been suckling at the mother's breast. The baby was perfect.

Later, I was completing the paperwork and had to pause and sit back. Reflecting on what happened in the ER that day: life, death, tragedy, and joy. Trying to find some special meaning or insight, it was difficult to comprehend. Doesn't matter what happens, the world goes on.

———————————————

It was 6 PM, and I'd just started my evening shift. "Dr. Thomson, we need you in the break room," someone hollered urgently. I thought this could be a prank, except for the urgency in the voice. I stepped in to find Phillip, an environmental service employee, laying on the floor. I knew him well, having worked together at our small ER over 10 years. His legs were elevated on a chair. Two PAs were kneeling beside him. "Did you hurt your back," I asked? Then I noticed he was quite pale, clammy, and slow to speak.

"I….I had a few spells the last few days. Like I might pass out."

The PA's said they had entered just before me and found him on the floor.

"Are you having any pain," I asked, while checking his pulse.

"No, just lightheaded. My heart is fluttering."

"Let's get a bed. His pulse is irregular and fast, maybe 200," I said. Other team members from the ER arrived and we lifted him onto the bed, swiftly moving two doors down the hall and into resuscitation room 2. Routine activity took over. He was undressed and placed in a gown, oxygen and cardiac monitors applied, two IVs were started. I quickly examined him. Pulse ox was 99 %, blood pressure 100 / 80, conjunctiva pink, lungs clear, no respiratory distress, heart tones normal, abdomen soft, and brief neurologic exam without any focal findings. I knew he was about 50-years-old. He had no other symptoms and no history of any medical problems.

My partner Dr. Michael Lincoln stepped in after hearing the commotion. Just then a strange, fast irregular heart rhythm about 200 beats per minute appeared on the cardiac monitor. "That's Torsades, or V tach," I said. "He needs cardioversion," Mike and I said simultaneously. Phillip's pulse was thready. He was passing out. We tried a synchronized shock at 100 Joules. It worked. Back to NSR, heart rate was 100. Phillip semiconscious, moaned in agony. A bolus of 150 mg of amiodarone (an antiarrhythmic) was pushed through the IV line. An ECG was done, no cardiac ischemia, it was normal. The QT (a space on the ECG) interval was normal as well. The monitor showed intermittent 3 to 10 beat runs of V tach. "Oh….There's a longer run. Shock him again. Same 100 Joules, I said.

"No, no, don't," Phillip cried out, he had woken up a bit. We paused for a few seconds, the V tach persisted, his pulse weak. He was pale and diaphoretic.

"Cardiovert him," I instructed the nurses. They shocked him for the second time. He moaned in discomfort. His heart rhythm converted back to NSR. We gave another bolus of amiodarone 150mg and started a drip. A few anxious minutes passed. We gave IV Versed for anxiety and sedation.

"Call the on-call Cardiologist." The V tach reappeared. Phillip was sleepy, semiconscious. We tried a synchronized shock with 200 Joules, it worked for only 30 seconds. "Give a bolus of lidocaine." Shocked again at 200 Joules. NSR seemed to hold a bit, but still the occasional runs of V tach. We hung procainamide. Dr. Faulkner Cardiology, called back. He was still in the hospital reading stress tests and echocardiograms. "I'll come right down; I'll be there in 3 minutes."

We gave 2 grams of magnesium IV push, and one bolus of IV fluids. Dr. Faulkner arrived just as we were doing another cardioversion. Back to the NSR. I told the story to Dr. Faulkner. He examined Phillip and reviewed the ECG and watched the HR monitor. Still the recurrent brief runs of V tach. He dialed the cell phone number of his partner, an electrophysiologist (a cardiologist who specializes in heart arrhythmias. Another long run of V tach. Another cardioversion. Repeat the amiodarone bolus was the recommendation.

"We've given 300 mg already," I said.

"Give another 300 mg," was the order. We repeated the amiodarone, and the magnesium. Then tried a beta-blocker. The medications didn't seem to have any effect. More runs of V tach, followed by more cardioversion. We had tried everything. I looked at the Cardiologist. He was anxious and perspiring heavily. I became concerned. We had run out of options. I realized that happened to me in critical situations. When nothing was working, and there were no more options, I would start to panic and break into a sweat.

Then suddenly (for no apparent reason) the arrhythmias disappeared. We had given double doses antiarrhythmics, they had been on board for quite a while. Maybe they finally began to work. We watched the heart monitor for a long time. No more V tach. Phillip rested peacefully with the sedative medication. He was out of immediate danger. He was admitted and transferred to the CCU.

About a week later, Phillip stopped by the ER. He said the doctors had run every test they could think of cardiac catheterization, MRI, even a heart biopsy. They inserted an ICD (an implantable cardioverter-defibrillator). The biopsy revealed cardiac sarcoidosis, a rare immune disorder of unknown etiology. He was on cardiac medication and the fainting spells had stopped. He thanked me profusely. "Thanks Phillip, but I can't take all the credit. My partner Dr. Michael Lincoln came into the resuscitation room and stayed the whole time. Two cardiologists were involved, and the ER staff performed fabulously. "The whole team saved your life."

15 Year Olds

"Go ahead James, tell the doctor what happened," instructed his mother.

"Well," the young man said slowly, "I picked a fight and I lost."

I liked James immediately. He was my first and only patient in my entire ER career to admit two things. First: picking a fight, and second: losing a fight. I treated hundreds of patients involved in physical altercations (mostly men, but many women as well) and never heard this before. The typical claims were: "I was minding my own business watching TV, I was waiting at the bus stop, I got sucker punched, I was breaking up the fight, there were four of them and they finally got the best of me."

James had been punched repeatedly in the face. He complained of pain, swelling and blood in the left eye. He denied other injuries. On exam there were small ecchymotic lumps over the forehead, orbits, zygomas (cheekbones), and left eyelids. His facial bones had no crepitus or deformity (indicating no fractures). His visual acuity and eye exam were normal except for bright red blood under the conjunctival membrane surrounding his left iris. This dramatic discoloration is concerning to patients and family, but fortunately is harmless. It turns black and purplish blue in a few days, then slowly yellowish brown. It takes two weeks to resolve completely.

We had a brief talk about subconjunctival hemorrhage, and a longer discussion about avoiding altercations and de-escalating conflict. I said to James, "It was refreshing to hear your honesty. It takes courage to admit a mistake. That will take you a long way."

"Hi Kelly, I'm Dr. Thomson. Tell me what happened." She was in our ENT chair, her mother seated off to one side. "I was eating popcorn and a kernel got stuck in my throat. You won't be able to get it out," she declared emphatically. Her mother perked her head up. How could Kelly know that? Posterior pharyngeal foreign bodies are common (fishbones, popcorn pieces, etc) and after many years it was routine for me to remove them.

"Oh, well, I'll take a look in a minute. Can you tell me where you can feel it stuck?" She pointed to the right tonsillar region below the angle of the mandible (lower jawbone).

After donning a headlight, I asked Kelly to open her mouth, and gently depressed her tongue with a wooden blade. A small piece of a popcorn kernel was wedged in the folds of the top portion of her right tonsil. "I can see the kernel, it's in the top of your right tonsil."

Kelly seemed unhappy and frowning said, "Well. You won't be able to get it out!" Her mother was aghast at her daughter's brashness.

I said, "It shouldn't be too difficult, it is easily visible. I have done it numerous times." Kelly was not impressed and glared at me with obvious hostility. I explained the straightforward procedure to her. "After spraying the area with a topical anesthetic, I want you to gargle for a few seconds. Then I will grasp the kernel with alligator forceps (that have a small jaw on the front). You may want to spit out the extra anesthetic, it tastes bitter.

139

"I never spit!" my young patient replied indignantly.

"Ok. Open your mouth and hold your breath." I sprayed the right tonsil thoroughly with topical Benzocaine. Kelly immediately began gagging profusely, then sat forward and vigorously spit out as much anesthetic solution as possible. "Open your mouth again. Take a deep breath and say Ahhhh." On the first attempt, in just a few seconds I was able to grasp the kernel. "Got it," I reported, holding it up for all to see. Kelly seemed genuinely shocked and said nothing. I took a second look to ensure complete removal and no additional foreign bodies.

"Thank the doctor," Kelly's mother insisted. Kelly looked at the floor and whispered, "Thanks."

When preparing the discharge instructions, I noted they lived in the same small town as my family. Returning to the ENT room I asked, "Do you go to Northville High School? You must know my son Matt or daughter Natalie."

Kelly replied, "Yes," remained expressionless, and didn't elaborate.

I didn't discuss many cases with my family. Arriving home that night I asked my wife Angela, "Do you know a girl Kelly Anderson or her family?"

She perked her head up "Why do you ask?"

"I treated Kelly for a minor problem and was able to take care of it in the ER. I asked her if she knew Natalie. She seemed stiff."

"Oh my goodness. You know all those cliques in high school? The one that Kelly is in, they hate Natalie! She would know that you're Natalie's dad."

———————————————

John presented in obvious distress. He had severe pain with swallowing and would occasionally spit up saliva. His airway was clear, no stridor or hoarseness. "What happened?" I asked.

"My girlfriend and I were having an argument. She was mad at me and said I didn't love her. I told her, I love you, I love you. She said if you love me, you'll eat this, and handed me her barrette. So, I swallowed it. Now it feels stuck right here," pointing under his sternal notch (a common location for esophageal foreign bodies to lodge).

"A lot of us have been there," I admitted (willing to do anything for the woman we loved). John's exam was otherwise normal. Nothing visible in the oral cavity, no palpable swelling in the neck, and lungs clear to auscultation. "I will notify our on-call gastroenterology team. The barrette must be removed before it erodes a hole through the esophageal wall."

Thirty minutes later John was whisked to the endoscopy suite. He was given IV Propofol (a sedative medication). A flexible scope was inserted down his throat and into the esophagus to allow the gastroenterologist to visualize and grasp the foreign body for removal. John tolerated the procedure well and was brought back to the ER for recovery. Sixty minutes later he was alert and ready for discharge.

"How are you feeling?" I asked.

"Okay," he replied forlornly. He had no pain and could swallow liquids well, but he didn't look happy.

"Did they give you the barrette?" I inquired.

"They offered it to me, but I didn't want it."

"Why not? Your girlfriend might like it."

"I don't care about the barrette. After I swallowed it, she broke up with me."

Complaints

Most patient complaints we received involved prolonged waiting times. Most of these were legitimate (and reflect a nationwide problem). The number of ER staff (physicians, nurses, technicians) scheduled throughout the day dependent upon the expected patient volume. This applies to the staffing of ancillary services (Laboratory, Radiology, Surgery, Inpatient Units, etc) as well. With variable numbers of patients arriving each day (as well as variable patient acuity) appropriate scheduling is a tremendous challenge. No hospital could afford to staff the ER for what would be the busiest day of the year. The result is that on busy days (I'd guess 20 percent of the time) the ER is understaffed and prolonged delays result.

When the hospital is full, admitted patients in the ER have to wait. This is common. Dramatic pictures of patients in beds, crammed along every hallway are shown in every article about ER overcrowding. The staff continue to care for them, as well as all the incoming ER patients. Most complaints are from patients with minor trauma or less severe medical issues. Of course, critically, and seriously ill patients are seen immediately, the other patients must wait. One recommended solution was to keep the waiting patients (and their families and friends) well informed of the situation, by circulating around the department regularly. I found this to be impossible. How could we take the time to step away from caring for critical patients every 30 or 40 minutes? There was no way.

The ER visit could not have been smoother. The 39-year-old man had been playing basketball and fell awkwardly. He injured his left shoulder and was in tremendous pain. His buddies lifted him carefully into their vehicle and came to our ER. I'd seen him being placed in a room, and immediately walked over. The patient was holding his left wrist with his right hand, in order to avoid any movement of his left shoulder. I asked, "Any other injuries? Any other pain? Any numbness or weakness?"

"No, no, no. Please hurry Doc, my shoulder is killing me," he begged.

After a brief general exam (to ensure no occult head, neck, or other injuries), I gently examined and palpated his left upper extremity and shoulder. He had a good left radial pulse, no loss of sensation, and good motor function of the left hand and wrist. There was mild fullness (swelling) of the anterior left shoulder and no bony tenderness or crepitus (grating sensation of fractured bone).

He had an anterior dislocation of the shoulder. A common injury that occurs when the arm is forcefully pulled up and back, during a hard fall. This force results in the humeral head (the proximal upper arm bone) moving forward (anterior) out of the socket (glenoid fossa, the lateral portion of the shoulder blade). It is immensely painful; any motion of a dislocated shoulder causes excruciating discomfort.

Joint reductions are a common procedure for ER physicians. I had performed close to a hundred. Early on, the techniques for reducing a dislocated shoulder required extensive pulling on the arm. Patients would typically scream in agony, even if given parental IV or IM (intramuscular) analgesic or sedative medications. Over the years many improved and effective techniques were developed. They were described in detail in the medical literature. I adopted many of them. Scapular (shoulder blade) rotation and the Spaso techniques were my favorites. Later I added a 20 cc injection of lidocaine into the shoulder joint for anesthesia (pain control) if an initial gentle reduction attempt failed.

In this case I tried the Spaso technique, and had the patient lay on his back on the ER bed. I gently took his wrist with my left hand and said, "We'll get you more comfortable." I held the arm very still. "Take really slow, deep breaths in and out." This should just take a minute or two. I'll hold your arm up." I applied gentle traction. After a minute, I could see him relax, and applied a little more traction. "Keep breathing slowly, relax…relax." I rotated his wrist externally a fraction. There was a "Thunk." I felt a bump and could see the anterior fullness disappear as his shoulder reduced.

"Aaaaaaaah," he said, "That feels so much better."

He'd been in the ER for about 10 minutes. We hadn't given any medication. Getting the patient to relax was the key. That allowed the head of the humerus to roll over the edge of the glenoid rim and back into position. "I think your dislocation is gone. We'll get an X-ray to confirm." We placed him in a shoulder immobilizer, a sling with a belt loop around the back. This is for comfort, and also keeps the hand by the belly button (which effectively prevents a redislocation). The X-rays were normal. He was discharged with routine instructions.

A month later I was shown a complaint letter from this gentleman. It wasn't about the care, but about the bill. The total charge for his

ER visit was $900 dollars; including the hospital portion, radiology charge and the physician fee. He seemed most upset about the physician fee, which was $200. He wrote: "Dr. Thomson was in the room with me for about 10 minutes. That comes to $1,200 per hour." He noted, "I'm an attorney, and $1,200 dollars per hour is completely unreasonable."

Our billing company wanted me to respond. I thought for a moment. He was correct about the ten minutes I'd spent with him. My care and treatment had been not just good, but phenomenal. The shoulder reduction only took about five minutes. I wrote him back. "The physician fee for all anterior shoulder reductions is $200, no matter what technique is used. Many physicians are not familiar with and have not mastered the newer techniques. Most patients wait with horrible pain, for an IV. Then wait for an X-ray to confirm the dislocation. Many reductions take 30 to 60 minutes. The doctor pulls with tremendous force, often repeatedly. The patient screams in agony each time, even with IV pain medication.

I saw you immediately upon your arrival. I was able to reduce your dislocation in a few minutes with minimal discomfort. My care and treatment were excellent and worth every penny of the $200. Please send in whatever amount you think is appropriate. Thank you."

———————————————

"That doctor's a racist." I picked my head up. I was at the workstation entering multiple orders and asking the unit tech to page the Intensivist for an admission. Looking over, I saw a young Black woman. She was upset, pointing in my direction. I turned and checked behind me, expecting another physician to be standing there. No, only me.

"Oh, what's the trouble?" I asked.

"We've been here almost two hours. You're taking everyone else ahead of my aunt because we're Black," she said adamantly. Everyone within earshot was staring at me.

I asked, "What room is your aunt in?"

"Right here," she said, gesturing behind her to room 12. I glanced at the chart rack. Number 12 was the next in line.

It had been a routine morning until the last 90 minutes. Two critically ill patients arrived simultaneously. An elderly man with obvious sepsis, and a woman with severe CHF causing respiratory failure. I'd just intubated the woman. The ER saw about 30,000 patients a year, approximately 80 to 90 per day. We had single physician coverage until noon. It was 11 AM.

"Your aunt is the next patient in line. I've been tied up with two critical patients. I can see her in about five minutes," I explained.

"We'll be leaving by then," she stated, and disappeared into room 12. I turned back and finished my admission orders. It took about five minutes. No one had ever accused me of being racist before, I was taken by surprise. I hadn't seen any Black patients or family in the ER that morning, so I was sure I hadn't discriminated against them. The ER was located in a rural area about 35 miles northwest of Detroit. About five percent of the patients we'd see were Black.

One of the great things about an ER is that all patients are equal. Doesn't matter who you are: rich or poor, young, or old, man or woman, insured or not. Religion, skin color, nationality, language spoken, does not matter. What matters in the ER is just how ill you are. Patients are seen according to their VS and how sick they appear. Patients are seen in a triage area by an experienced RN. If seriously or critically ill, they are immediately brought to a bed inside the ER. If the patient is stable, they are placed into an open bed or back out to the waiting area if no beds are available. A clerical staff person would then start a chart. Patients from the waiting room are brought to the back according to their time of arrival.

It is well known that people can and often do have subconscious bias. We'd had courses highlighting those issues (in areas of age, appearance, education etc.) I am certain I have some. I tried to recognize possible areas of bias and do my best to eliminate it.

Entering room 12 I introduced myself. There was a middle-aged Black woman in the bed, her niece in the chair next to her. A quick review of the triage note revealed stable VS. I apologized for the wait, "I was caring for two critically ill patients."

"You took care of them before my aunt," the niece stated directly.

"Well yes. But we must see critical patients first," I replied.

"You took other people ahead of us. We're Black, so you made us wait," she persisted.

"Well, I didn't know the color of your skin. The door to your room was closed and I didn't see you come in. Also, all the patients in the ER and the waiting room had to wait." There was an awkward, silent pause. The niece wasn't convinced.

I could have kept explaining, but in my experience if my first one or two points don't sway the patient or family, then the next few certainly won't either. Besides, the ER was still busy. There were four additional charts in the rack. "At this time, I think there are three options. I can see your aunt as a patient, you could wait another 50 minutes until the next physician arrives, or you can sign out and go to another ER."

Another long pause, they looked at each other. The aunt spoke up, "It's Ok, you can be my doctor." They allowed me to perform a history and physical examination. She had been having episodic RUQ abdominal pain; careful palpation of that area revealed no tenderness. I ordered numerous blood tests and an ultrasound study of her GB (gallbladder). The laboratory tests were normal. The ultrasound identified numerous large gallstones, but no inflammation or edema of the GB wall. She was stable and didn't require admission or immediate surgery. We were able to schedule an appointment with a GS (general surgeon) in a few days.

At the end of my shift one of the nurses caught up with me and asked, "Didn't that make you mad, when they called you racist?"

"No, I was too surprised. Actually, I felt sad."

"Why is that? she asked.

I thought a bit. "I bet they've been made to wait many times. Now, when something unfair happens they assume it's discrimination."

I had minor personal experience with bias, certainly on a different scale. I was the shortest person in school until junior year. I'd gotten bullied a fair amount, mostly verbal. Oddly, the worst offenders were the smaller boys (but still bigger than me). I didn't like it one bit and couldn't do much about it. The bullying resolved when I had a growth spurt. "Could you imagine having to go through life and through no fault of your own be held back by something you have no control over? You can't fix it, and it never ends. That would be terribly frustrating. That's what makes me sad."

Welcome to Jackson

It was October 15th, 2008, my first shift in Jackson. Our company was taking over the physician staffing in the ER at Allegiance Health, the only hospital in Jackson County, Michigan. There would be two months of overlap as physicians from both groups would take shifts. All the ER physicians worked from a central location "The Fishbowl," a large room with glass walls located behind the main nurses' station near the EMS entrance. The proximity allowed for effective communication. This was a busy ER with three or four physicians working at one time to handle the large volume.

An EMS radio call came into the nursing station. "This is alpha 112. We are bringing a morbidly obese male, over 500 lbs., with lethargy and difficulty breathing. Two attempts at intubation failed. We are providing BVM ventilation, the pulse ox is 86%. ETA (estimated time of arrival) is five minutes."

Kathy the charge RN replied, "Bring him to Room 1 (Resuscitation). She called for respiratory therapy and notified the ER critical care team to prepare for the patient's arrival.

I was in the fishbowl at my computer station. So were two other physicians, both from the prior physician group. We could easily hear the EMS report. Typically, physicians would take turns (or whomever was most available) caring for an incoming critical patient. It had been a slow morning so any of us could accept the new patient. We had a couple minutes to tidy up any loose ends. The other physicians scurried off. I waited at the main nurses' station.

Four minutes later, EMS burst through the entrance with a massive individual on their cart. He weighed well over 500 lbs. and was in critical condition. The patient was unresponsive and dusky in color. The paramedics were attempting to ventilate him by BVM. BVM can ventilate patients beautifully but may be extremely challenging and ineffective in morbidly obese individuals. It's difficult to get a good fit over the patient's mouth and nose. Even more challenging when a man has a thick beard. If the airway is partially obstructed by the large tongue, swollen soft palate and pharyngeal tissue, then good ventilation is nearly impossible. Frequently an ET tube is required. ER physicians (and Anesthesiologists) know this can be a nightmare. If a secure airway tube cannot be inserted, death is likely. The EMS crew raced a few steps to the Resuscitation room. I glanced around, the other physicians were nowhere in sight. It was up to me, the new guy.

Room 1 was packed with about 16 people. The ER critical care team and two respiratory therapists were there (and about 10 interested observers). Simultaneously the patient was attached to monitors, two good IV lines established, and two respiratory therapists worked together trying BVM ventilation. I listened to a brief report from the paramedics while quickly examining the patient. His chest wall was massively obese. I couldn't hear any breath sounds through all the adipose tissue. I checked the monitors and the BVM ventilation attempts. He had a large coarse beard, and the face mask fit was poor. The pulse oxygen reading hovered around 80 %. This man could have a cardiac arrest at any moment. He required a good airway immediately.

"Let's intubate him," I said. I asked them to call anesthesiology down, and to bring their fiberoptic scope (a new piece of equipment, and they kept the only one).

They responded, "We can be down in 20 minutes."

The largest patient I had ever intubated was a man weighing about 380 lbs. There is so much swollen tissue including the tongue, soft palate, throat, and neck being able to see the vocal cords (the entrance to the trachea and lungs) is tremendously difficult. You could blindly pass a tube down the throat, but entering the trachea was rarely successful.

In most patients the backup airway is an incision in the anterior neck. Dissecting quickly down to the tracheal region, then cutting through the cricothyroid membrane and inserting a tube into the trachea. In a morbidly obese patient, with 8 to 10 inches of fatty tissue in this region, the surgical airway is a hopeless task. There was no other option, I had to try oral intubation.

Fortunately, we had good IV access. I ordered 300 mg of succinylcholine. We continued BVM ventilation. In about 45 seconds we saw a few fasciculations; after a few more seconds he was paralyzed. The patient's head was elevated about 30 degrees. I had an assistant tilt the head back slightly. I stood on a foot stool for elevation and inserted a straight bladed laryngoscope and tried to find the vocal cords. I couldn't see them. I suctioned some secretions and looked again. I could see a small opening at the top of my visual field. On both sides were small bumps, the arytenoid cartilages. This was the lowest part of the opening between the vocal cords. I advanced the ET tube (I had placed a malleable stylet inside and bent it upward at an angle). The tip of the ET tube

153

was in front of the opening, but now obscured my view. I pushed it forward a few centimeters, then removed the stylet. "I think it's in." We attached the bag to the proximal end of the ET tube and started ventilation. The inline CO_2 detector was changing color from yellow to purple. The ET tube was in the trachea! I gripped the tube tightly. It could easily become dislodged, and I didn't want to do that again. The respiratory therapists took over. They taped the ET securely and attached it to a ventilator. The critical danger was over.

I looked up. The entire intubation procedure had taken a couple of minutes. The room was filled with people. Nobody said a word. I was shocked. This was at the very least a small miracle. I had just smoothly intubated a massively obese man, on the very first attempt! Certainly, one of my best lifesaving interventions ever. At my ER in Novi there would have been a fair bit of praise and joyful hollering. I left the room thinking: "This is a tough crowd. Here in Jackson, I don't know, maybe this happens all the time."

A bit later, when there was a lull, I tracked down and asked the charge nurse Kathy, "What happened in Room 1?"

"What do you mean?" she answered back.

"That was probably my best intubation ever, and no one said a word."

 "Come with me," she motioned over to a quiet corner. "You know your two hot shot partners that started here last week? Well, they're walking around here like they can walk on water. Worse yet, they made some cutting remarks to the nurses about the previous doctors. Many of the nurses are good friends with those physicians, having worked alongside them for years. Our ER staff like and respect them a great deal. So, they didn't take kindly to those comments. They all piled into the resuscitation to see the action. They knew the patient was about to crash, and that the intubation could be a nightmare. Don't worry, they were impressed. It's just that they were hoping you might struggle a bit." The light bulb was coming on. I had noticed the frosty reception when being introduced that morning. I had chalked it up to a busy place and everyone working hard and going about their own business.

"Wow. Kathy, thanks for clueing me in."

"Dr. Kirshner, have you ever amputated a patient's arm?"

I had just seen a 67-year-old woman who had been to the Jackson ER the evening before. She had been in good health and dropped a book from a shelf that landed on the top of her left wrist three days prior. Yesterday morning the mildly swollen and bruised area became unbearably painful. One of my partners saw her, obtained an X-ray (normal), and gave one IM injection of morphine. She was discharged with stable VS. This morning her husband found her confused, weak, with a fever and brought her back to the ER.

Her past history was unremarkable, no serious medical problems. On general appearance she was occasionally moaning, confused, her skin cool and clammy. VS: 100-degree temp, RR of 20, HR of

128 and BP 90 / 60. Likely early septic shock. The only abnormality on her exam was her left arm. There was a small bruise on the top of the wrist with mild diffuse slightly warm and pink swelling extending halfway up to her elbow. The skin was intact, no abrasion or laceration. Gentle ROM of her left wrist and fingers was normal and didn't seem to cause any discomfort (ruling out joint or tendon sheath infections).

What was unusual was palpation of the swelling. There was no crepitus or subcutaneous air (signs of abscess). Instead, I found a "squishy" sensation from soft edema fluid under the skin and above the muscle compartment. The only likely diagnosis was necrotizing fasciitis (flesh eating bacteria). This is a rare and highly fatal bacterial infection, usually resistant to antibiotics. The only treatment to possibly save her life would be a fasciotomy (surgically open the fascial compartments) of the arm or amputation.

Dr. Kirshner general surgery had returned my call. "This is Mark Thomson, one of the new ER doctors. I have a lady with necrotizing fasciitis. I think she needs an immediate fasciotomy or left arm amputation. Have you ever amputated an arm before?"

"No, and I'm not doing one today. I'm about to start a hemi-colectomy (remove half a patient's colon). Why don't you order a CT scan and I'll see her when I'm finished?"

"I'll have to transfer her to the trauma center. I don't think it can wait, and as you know CT scans often don't identify necrotizing fasciitis well." I walked back to the patient's room while talking to Dr. Kirshner.

"How do you know it's necrotizing fasciitis?" he asked.

"I'm not 100 percent sure, but nothing else is likely. I just noticed the swelling is now at her elbow, and she's only been in the ER for 30 minutes. The infection is rapidly ascending." He asked me to send her to the trauma center.

I went to the physician work room, entered orders, and paged the trauma center and helicopter transfer service. I doubted the patient would survive. Just then, Dr. Kirshner walked quickly towards the patient room. He decided to have a look himself. I tagged along. He stayed in the room for two minutes, asking a few questions, but most of that time carefully examining and palpating the left arm. "We'll take her," he pronounced. Minutes later the patient was transferred to the OR.

I followed the patient's admission through her medical record and talked to Dr. Kirshner. He had to amputate the whole arm when they found signs of significant infection already to the patient's axilla (armpit). Post Op she developed septic shock and had a stormy 14 day stay in the ICU. She survived but was quite weak and debilitated. She was discharged to a rehab facility and was expected to recover.

I was impressed with Dr. Kirshner. I was new to Jackson and had never met him. Over the phone he was hesitant to believe the strange ER doctor's clinical diagnosis of necrotizing fasciitis (which is very rare). It would have been much easier to continue with his elective surgical case. He decided to operate immediately on just his clinical diagnosis (no confirmatory testing), and then perform an arm amputation for the first time. His decisions and actions saved the patient's life.

Customer Service

Years before the end of my career hospitals began to adapt many business practices in the provision of health care services. I was hesitant to adopt a business model. As far as I knew, the goal of most businesses was to make money. My goal in the ER was to provide world class health care to those in need. Of course, the ER and the hospital needed to pay bills and keep the doors open. We needed to be cost efficient and productive. I am certain that using business principles and methods to improve our hospital and ER services was well intentioned and resulted in a fair amount of success. I am also certain there were unintended consequences.

One business process that was adopted by hospitals nationwide (required by Medicare and other large insurance companies) was "Customer Service." I understood the concept, and it was important for many businesses (thinking Starbucks, Panera Bread, Target, Kroger, etc). I was hesitant to embrace this notion in providing health care. Certainly, patients that are happy with their physician's advice were more likely to follow it. But customer service in the ER, in the relationship between physician and patient was more complex. I had to advise many patients to change their lifestyle habits (quit smoking, quit drinking, exercise, lose weight, take your medications, don't use drugs, follow safe sex guidelines, store your gun safely, etc). If anyone believes that I had enough time to counsel patients with these problems, and have them be happy about it, they had not spent much time in my ER.

Part of the customer service process for the ER was to send questionnaires to discharged patients (admitted patients would receive an inpatient survey). The patient would rate various aspects of their ER visit including how happy they were with the physician. We would be rated on a one to five scale with five the best score. Medicare and the major insurance companies began to hold back a portion of their payments, keeping the funds in a pool for distribution. Hospitals and physicians would receive a portion of the funds depending upon how they were rated by, "Customers."

For hospitals the amount of money involved was eye opening, in the multimillion-dollar range. In just a few years, physician incentive programs were initiated. Rewarding those physicians with high rating scores a significant bonus. I was incensed. I had dedicated my entire education and training learning how to provide up to date world class medical care. There were few proven benefits to patients' health from these programs. After 30 years of practicing in the ER would I have to concentrate on customer service? I had more important things to think about, such as: when to consider a life threatening infection in an infant; what antibiotics were best for an immunosuppressed pregnant woman with pneumonia; did the elderly patient with shortness of breath have only an exacerbation of COPD (Chronic Obstructive Pulmonary Disease / Smokers Lung) or was there an additional possibility of a pulmonary embolism; should I order a CT angiogram on the anxious young woman with a slightly unusual headache? Critical decisions like these needed to be made on almost every shift.

I was called into the administrative office to review my customer service score. Dr. Cynthia Harris (my supervising physician) said, "Your score is 4.37 (out of 5)." Not bad, but I was below the cut off and I would miss out on the bonus.

"It's okay, I don't care. I'm not changing my practice," I said stubbornly.

"Come on Mark, it's important," she replied.

"Not to me."

"Well, it is to the hospital, and to our physician group. To keep our ER contract, we must maintain a high customer service score. Many of your scores were five, but also a few one's and two's. Let's look at a few of your low score cases," she suggested.

I already suspected where these low ratings were coming from. Reviewing the charts confirmed two common themes. Patients unhappy that I hadn't given them opiates, and patients with minor illness or injury that had long stays in the ER. I was particularly stubborn with patients that would present with a feigned illness and wanting pain medication. I would tell them directly they had an opiate addiction or opioid use disorder and would never give them opiate medication or a Rx. She suggested writing "Opioid Use Disorder" as the first diagnosis on the patient's chart, then their survey would be thrown out. I had never done that, not wanting to "label" a patient. My routine was to list that diagnosis last.

I also could be short with patients who presented with minor problems and wanted to be taken ahead of others. When I first started in the ER nearly all patients were quite understanding about nurses and physicians caring for the sickest patients first. This empathetic awareness seemed to disappear over the same time "Customer service" became the important mantra. More than once I spoke abruptly to a patient when it was obvious the ER was extremely busy, and I was taking care of a critically ill patient.

I would be walking to the workstation, they would interrupt and ask, "Hey Doc, won't you just check my foot X-ray?"

My usual stern response was, "No. You have to wait your turn, just like everyone else." I never added, "You selfish, inconsiderate jerk." I knew better than to say that. However, my tone of voice and body language certainly did.

———————————

A 37-year-old man presented to the ER with severe chest pain. He was anxious, hyperventilating, and screaming in discomfort. He told the triage nurse, "My pain is 15 (out of 10), just like my previous pulmonary embolism." He claimed to have had 13 prior blood clots in his lungs. She brought him directly to our resuscitation room, checked his VS and asked me to see him. He repeated this history and said he needed pain medication; the pain was unbearable.

I was immediately suspicious. I had never read of a patient with more than three episodes of pulmonary emboli. Also, they cause chest pain, but typically not extremely severe. Also, his heart rate was 96 and oxygenation was 100 %, both normal (and would be extremely unusual in any patient with a symptomatic blood clot in their lung). I swiftly completed his exam, it was normal. I told the patient we would start with some tests, give him some non-narcotic pain medicine through the IV, and I would check his medical record.

He became agitated and started hollering, "I need pain medicine. They gave me Dilaudid last time. I can't wait. I can't wait!"

I told him, "I must check your medical record on the computer. I'll be back in a few minutes."

Reviewing the medical record, he had been to our ER twice within the last two months. Two CT angiograms with contrast were performed, they were normal. There were no pulmonary emboli. I went back to see him. He had ripped his IV out. Blood was dripping down his arm. He knew what was coming. I said I would be happy to evaluate him, to try and help with his discomfort.

"You won't give me any strong pain medicine?" he asked.

"Not unless I find any pathology. Your last two CT scans were normal."

He walked out of the ER, not waiting for a dressing of the IV site. He screamed, "I'm not paying your bill. You'll be hearing from my attorney." These threats have no effect on ER physicians. Approximately 33 percent of our patients cannot pay our bills (most are poor and have no insurance). Attorneys do not file lawsuits against physicians in these types of cases.

I looked further into his medical record. Two of my partners had seen him. I was perplexed. During the first visit he complained of severe chest pain and had received a two mg dose of Dilaudid IV push, a powerful opiate medication. He had a complete work up with blood tests, ECG, and a CT angiogram. All were negative. No embolism and no pathology. The listed diagnosis was, "Chest Pain." Despite that he was given a Rx at discharge for 20 powerful opiate pain tablets.

He returned (not a surprise) four weeks later. At this ER visit he had similar complaints. He again received two mg of Dilaudid IV push, and another complete work up was performed, including another CT angiogram. All tests were perfectly normal. Despite this he received another two mg dose of Dilaudid IVP. His diagnosis again was, "Chest Pain." He was given a Rx, this time for 30 of the powerful opiate tablets. This was about the most obvious case of opiate addiction and drug seeking I had ever seen.

Why had two physicians given him large doses of opiate medication? I suspected that the customer service program had something to do with it. It takes time and significant emotional energy to confront these patients. Their response is often hostile and aggressive. It is much easier to give one or two doses of IV medication and write a Rx. I finished documenting the medical record. For the first time in my career, I listed the primary diagnosis: "Opioid Use Disorder."

———————————

Dr. Jeff Robinson, Chairperson of Pediatrics was on the telephone. "Mark, I need you to review a case. Dr. Winters (James Winters was one of my partners) admitted a young child yesterday evening with RSV (respiratory syncytial virus) and completely missed DKA. It's a bad mistake. I'm concerned about his clinical judgment."

"The child didn't have RSV?" I asked. "Jim is a sharp guy, and usually on target," I mentioned.

"Oh, there was RSV. But he didn't run any lab tests beyond the nasal swab."

"Ok Jeff. Our department meeting is in two weeks. We'll review the case and I'll get back to you."

RSV is a virus that virtually every child is exposed to by the age of two. Only a small percent gets seriously ill, and about one percent have to be hospitalized. It is dangerous for premature infants with BPD (bronchopulmonary dysplasia or lung scarring). The virus causes inflammation in airways, especially the small airways (bronchiolitis). Symptoms are fever, cough, and wheezing. Treatment is supportive: fluids (if dehydration), oxygen and bronchodilators for bronchospasm and wheezing. There are no effective antiviral medications. Occasionally the bronchodilators don't work well, resulting in the need for admission. After a day or two most children recover uneventfully.

DKA is a severe complication of insulin dependent diabetes where the blood glucose gets high, and large amounts of glucose get excreted in the urine. Due to osmotic pressure a large amount of water and potassium gets excreted in the urine as well. Common symptoms include excessive thirst, excessive urination, nausea, vomiting, and abdominal pain. The resulting dehydration and electrolyte imbalance can be life threatening. DKA is hard to consider and diagnose if there is no history of diabetes. DKA in young children is often the first presentation of diabetes. It is commonly precipitated by an infection.

I pulled the chart. The case was a 14-month-old who had been perfectly healthy. There was no history of medical problems. No asthma or diabetes, no family history of asthma or diabetes. Two days prior to presentation he developed a low-grade fever, decreased appetite, cough and wheezing. There was no vomiting or abdominal pain, no note about increased thirst or urination. In the

ER he appeared ill but not critically. He had a fast RR (36) and HR (140). He was noted to have dry lips and oral mucous membranes. There were diffuse wheezes on chest auscultation. A nasal swab was positive for RSV. The child received three updraft treatments with bronchodilators and had minimal improvement. A chest X-ray was taken, no pneumonia was present. His RR and HR didn't improve. The diagnosis: RSV and persistent bronchospasm (wheezing).

The case was reviewed at our monthly department meeting. This meeting is attended by physicians and MLP's (mid-level providers, PAs, and NPs). Concerns were raised about the lack of documentation of ROS (review of systems, a list of many questions for patient symptoms). Admitted patients and many ill ER patients commonly have a thorough ROS. Many practitioners admitted abbreviating this process once an accurate diagnosis has been made that explains the patient's signs and symptoms. Note was made about recent studies that concluded that most children admitted with RSV undergo numerous tests. The test results are usually normal and thought to be unnecessary. Without a history of diabetes, excessive thirst, or urination no one would have ordered a blood sugar. The conclusions were: the child received good care, it was an excellent teaching case illustrating a hidden second diagnosis, and it emphasizes the importance of performing a thorough ROS.

As I prepared the case for review, I examined the care and treatment by the pediatricians during the hospital stay. The admitting night shift pediatrician performed an admitting history and exam. There was no ROS completed. His work up, care and treatment were nearly identical to the one documented in the ER by Dr. Winters. No additional tests were ordered. No DKA was diagnosed. The day shift pediatrician did another history and exam. No ROS was documented. Her work up, care and treatment were similar. Again, no tests were ordered and no DKA was diagnosed.

I discovered a nurse's note at 11:52 AM. "Child urinating frequently. Dipstick positive for glucose. Physician notified." This was the first notation of excessive thirst or urination. It appears that an astute nurse observed the abnormal urination and tested it herself (there was no order for the test). I suspect this child developed diabetes during the stress of his RSV infection. This caused a gradual increase in the blood glucose and resulted in increasing urination. The day shift RN deserved all the credit for considering and making the diagnosis.

I sent a summary note to Dr. Robinson. I called him as well and reviewed our conclusions with him. He was incredulous, "How could anyone miss the DKA!?"

I replied, "I think his diabetes and DKA were just developing at the time of his ER visit. We certainly emphasized the importance of doing a thorough ROS. That may have caught the excessive urination; if present."

Dr. Robinson wasn't mollified. "At the very least, I think your ER physician should have run some tests."

"Jeff, our whole department reviewed the case. I think you should present the case, including the work up performed by both the night and day shift pediatricians at your next department meeting. We stand by our doctor."

At some point a national consensus developed that doctors weren't treating patient's pain adequately. Articles appeared in medical journals (many supported by pharmaceutical companies) recommending opiate pain prescriptions and suggesting the risks of addiction were overstated. There were many stories documenting the agony of patients when not receiving adequate pain control. In the ERs where I worked, I wasn't sure that it was true. Pain was part of the chief complaint of most patients. The nurses and staff were compassionate and always concerned about relieving the patient's pain, readily notifying me if additional medication were needed. The biggest problem was delay. If the ER was swamped (a common occurrence) then getting pain medication timely to the suffering patient was a challenge. Physicians had been taught (and were concerned) about the dangers of over treating patient's pain and contributing to opiate addiction.

A new process was undertaken. The patient's "Pain Score" would be taken along with the VS. This pain score was a self-reporting score on a scale of 1 to 10 (10 being the most severe). It would be repeated as necessary throughout the ER stay and again at the time of discharge. The pain score became the fifth vital sign (along with temperature, HR, RR, and BP). Charts would be reviewed monthly. The initial and final pain scores were examined carefully. The goal was to ensure rapid and effective pain control, which should be easily documented by a significantly lower pain score at discharge. They would separate the scores out per individual physician. Of note, they did not tabulate how much oral or IV opiate medication was being used.

Many patients caught on quickly. They realized if they rated their headache or chest pain a "10" then they would be taken into the ER and not forced to wait. I began to see patients (usually younger ones) smiling and laughing while talking on their cell phones when entering their room. I'd have to double check the pain score, written as a "10." The "Pain Score" process remained throughout my career. It must have been one of the contributors to the "Opiate Crisis" a few years down the road.

We ensure patient comfort by numerous methods: covering them with a warm blanket, splinting the injured extremity, giving ibuprofen or acetaminophen. These measures provided good pain control, but often not dramatic. Many ER patients are evaluated and discharged in about two to three hours. If you want to make a difference in the pain score the easiest way is to give a large dose of oral or IV opiate pain medication. The use of opiate medication increased.

I was always concerned about the risk of contributing to a patient's addiction. My habit when prescribing pain medication was to write for a maximum of three days. Usually 12 to 20 pills, depending on how often they were to be taken. I never wrote for more than 20 tablets. Making it easy for me to reply "No" to the occasional call from a pharmacist when asked, "Did I really mean to Rx #120 pills?" Someone must have generously changed the number by adding a one in front of the 20. I began to write out the number, "Twenty" as well.

I used an observational pain assessment in every patient encounter. This includes watching facial expressions, listening to tone of voice and speech pattern, and observing body position. Pain is a subjective symptom, and self-reporting (pain score) is certainly important. If my pain assessment matched the patients reported Pain Score, I was confident in prescribing the correct amount of pain medication. If they were discrepant, I would order opiates cautiously.

A separate problem is addiction to opiates among health care providers. ER staff are similar to patients and have similar rates of drug abuse and addiction. I knew one physician and one nurse in our ER that were discovered diverting opiates (ordered for patients) to their own use. Both were given a second chance and allowed to return to work after finishing treatment programs. They both relapsed, and their employment terminated.

———————————————

One evening a 60-year -old woman presented with massive epistaxis (nose bleeding). Active bleeding can be challenging to control. One effective method is to cauterize the offending blood vessel by applying silver nitrate. To perform this, the physician needs to clearly see the actively bleeding vessel (difficult with massive bleeding). One solution is to apply liquid cocaine on a piece of cotton to the area and then pinch the nose. Cocaine is an excellent vasoconstrictor and topical anesthetic. The amount used is small. Patients do not get high.

I asked Vicki, the RN assisting, to bring cocaine (kept in a locked cabinet inside the locked medication room). After applying the cocaine, the patient's nasal bleeding decreased, and I was able to cauterize the vessel and stop the epistaxis.

169

When completing my procedure note in the medical record, I happened to review the nurse's note. Vicki was a diligent RN and thoroughly documented the patient condition, discharge VS, and details of the ER encounter. Her last sentence, "Cocaine used by Dr. Thomson," wasn't entirely accurate. Someone might interpret that I had taken the cocaine myself!

I asked Vicki to add a note about cocaine used for the patient. She added, "Cocaine used intranasally by Dr. Thomson." That still didn't seem right. I made her add, "Cocaine applied topically to the patient's nasal mucosa."

———————————

Another change that had unintended consequences was when ERs had beds separated by curtains and newly constructed or renovated ERs had private rooms. Privacy and comfort were the driving forces and are important considerations. Isolating patients however did just that, isolated patients. Loneliness, boredom, and focusing on one's own personal suffering often resulted. Patients in wards or on beds separated by curtains are in noisy areas with many distractions.

What I observed in those areas were conversations, shared stories, and understanding about the distress and misery of others. Empathy and compassion were commonplace. Patients obtained a unique perspective and intimate knowledge about injury and disease. This close personal experience imprints deeply into memory, in ways that reading a book, watching a movie or being on the internet cannot.

Imaging Advancements

I started my career in emergency medicine in 1982. For the first 20 years, our ER was a small free standing emergency department. There was single coverage with one emergency medicine physician. There was no backup. We saw all patients who came into the emergency department, and accepted EMS units (Ambulances). Patients that required hospital admission were transferred to nearby hospitals (15 to 30 minutes away). There were no surgeons available to help with procedures. No anesthesiologists for help with airway management. No OB / GYN physicians for precipitous deliveries. This allowed for broad practice opportunities, but also created many challenging and stressful moments.

I was always concerned a patient might present with pericardial tamponade. This is where fluid accumulates in the pericardial sac (around the heart) and develops pressure. Normally, the right side of the heart accepts venous blood under low pressure and pumps it through the lungs for oxygenation. This oxygenated blood returns to the left side of the heart and is pumped out with high pressure through the aorta to circulate through the body. In pericardial tamponade the accumulating fluid increases and creates pressure around the heart. This pressure decreases the venous blood return to the right side of the heart resulting in poor blood flow. This causes hypotension, shock, and then death.

Pericardiocentesis (where a large needle is inserted in the pericardial sac) to drain the fluid and relieve the pressure can be lifesaving. For many years this procedure was a "Blind" technique using anatomical landmarks. Pericardial tamponade is quite rare. Prior to US (ultrasound), the diagnosis was difficult to make in the

ER. Thinking about plunging a large bore needle deep towards the heart in an unstable patient with just a possibility of pericardial tamponade was anxiety provoking. However, pericardial effusion is easily diagnosed with ultrasound. US was not readily available in the emergency department for many years. The machines were bulky and expensive. Specially trained technicians did the scans. The images were interpreted by a radiologist, typically the next morning. This wouldn't be of any help for an unstable crashing patient in the emergency department. In a few years however, rapid technological improvements were made, and portable ultrasound machines became available and affordable.

Nowadays, all emergency medicine resident physicians are thoroughly trained on using portable US equipment. Years ago, I was on my own. I enthusiastically took two ultrasound courses to learn the basics of scanning and interpreting the ultrasound images. Once our emergency department purchased a portable ultrasound machine, I needed to improve my skills. I practiced on many willing patients. Taking a couple of minutes, I would perform multiple scans. I would start in the neck and identify the location of the jugular vein (later I'd use a similar US scan for guidance when inserting a large IV in that location). Proceeding to the heart, I would check the pericardial sac, contractility, and the cardiac chambers. Moving to the abdomen, I would scan the GB checking for gallstones and for fluid in Morrison's pouch (the perihepatic space). Then I would scan in the midline for the aorta looking for aneurysmal dilatation, then into the LUQ (left upper quadrant) to find the spleen. The kidneys and bladder were next. Scanning through the bladder in female patients I would image the uterus. Teaching myself, the learning curve was a long, slow process. With persistence, I gradually improved. Morbidly obese patients were especially difficult to scan and obtain good images. Due to the physics of ultrasound waves, the closer the transducing scanner was to the organ the sharper the images produced. Having patients turn on their side and / or take a deep breath could markedly improve the US image.

No question, this safe, non-invasive technology was a significant benefit for many patients. Before US arrived, much of my evaluation was done by careful palpation. I would gently press in different locations, furrow my brow, softly say "Hymmm," and then make an educated guess. Now, in just seconds, I could get a clear picture of the organ. Amazing.

In 2008 our physician group obtained the contract in the ER at the hospital in Jackson, Michigan. This was a busy place, seeing about 80,000 patients each year. We were able to start a residency program in Emergency Medicine, and help the ER become a Level I trauma center. Most shifts had two to three attending physicians working, as well as two to three residents. After 20 years of being the lone physician in my emergency department, working in Jackson was a refreshing change. The ability to have a quick discussion with superbly trained partners was exhilarating.

Dr. Nicholas Dyc was one of my new partners. His US skills were fantastic. His soft spoken, unassuming, and confident demeanor made him an excellent teacher. On my first shift working alongside him I asked, "Hey Nic, can you watch me do some US scanning and give me some tips?"

"Happy to," he chimed. My patient was stable and happy to allow me to scan away. I went through my repertoire: neck, heart, abdomen, etc. Within each area he'd make an insightful suggestion. For example: tip the US transducer a bit, and then immediately a beautiful image would appear on the screen. Nic pointed out the parasternal and long axis cardiac views. The best heart images I'd ever produced appeared. I always had difficulty imaging the spleen. Nic spotted the trouble, "It's more posterior; turn the patient over a bit more. Now have the patient inhale and hold their breath." A perfect picture of the spleen jumped onto the screen. Wow! My learning curve jumped.

I asked Nic, "Could you show me how to scan the heart for RV (Right Ventricle) collapse?"

"No problem, mate," he replied. RV collapse is a crucial finding in patients with fluid in their pericardial sac. It is a reliable sign of early pericardial tamponade. Going back to the parasternal cardiac view I found the RV. Nic pointed and said, "Look at this area of the RV; the wall. Keep your eye on it and watch carefully during diastole (the time when the heart rests and fills with blood). If this portion collapses instead of expanding, then there is tamponade. The patient needs emergency drainage."

Three months later, a young Black woman presented to my Novi ER about 10 PM on a Saturday evening with shortness of breath. She had been feeling poorly for about a week, mostly fatigued. No chest pain, cough, or fever, but she did notice short of breath with exertion for the last few days. The physical exam was unremarkable, except for her VS: RR 24, HR 112, and BP 90 / 60. I was concerned about the possibility of a pulmonary embolism, (a blood clot in the lungs). Black women have a higher risk of blood clots. If they traveled through the veins into the lungs the clots could block blood flow and cause sudden death.

I remembered about cardiac US for patients with hypotension (low blood pressure) or shock. She did not have shock but was tachycardic and the BP was low. Placing the US probe to the left of the sternum I easily visualized the heart. Oh! There was an obvious, large pericardial effusion. I hadn't expected that. Could it be under pressure? I stared for some time at the RV, watching the wall move throughout the cardiac cycle. The image would shift a bit, during the respiratory breathing cycle. Then, I could see it. The free muscular wall of the RV was collapsing during diastole. No doubt about it. She was "stable" for the moment, but if that pericardial fluid increased a bit, she could become critically unstable quickly. She needed pericardial drainage, soon.

I paged the on-call Cardiologist and cardiac cath lab team. The Cardiologist called back immediately, "What do you have Mark?"

"A young woman with a pericardial tamponade. She needs it drained," I explained

"Tonight? The cath team isn't in the hospital. They'd have to be called in," he replied.

"Well, she is tachycardic and has RV collapse on cardiac echo (US)," I answered.

"How'd you get the echo?" he asked. He knew that the cardiac echo technicians were only available during the day, Monday through Friday.

"I did it myself."

"Are you sure about the RV collapse?" he inquired.

I smiled, thinking about the instruction from Dr. Dyc. "Absolutely," I replied confidently. "I've already notified the cath team."

The patient was transferred to the Cath Lab. About 40 minutes later the Cardiologist stopped by the ER. "Hey Mark, you were right," he said. "We drained a fair amount of fluid and placed a pericardial catheter for continued drainage. Waiting until tomorrow morning would have been dangerous. Good call."

"Thanks, but one of my partners, Nic Dyc, deserves a lot of the credit. He recently showed me how to confirm the RV collapse." A few days later I saw the Cardiologist again. The young woman was about to be discharged. He told me her diagnosis was SLE (Lupus). The pericardial catheter was out, she was on medication. Her prognosis was excellent.

Another major technological improvement during my career in the ER was the development of the CT scanner. For many years the only CT scan we would use routinely was for the head / brain. With improvements in speed, rotation, table movement, and computer data processing the imaging capabilities were fantastic. CT scanning became a tremendous asset in patient evaluation. The drawbacks to CT scans are twofold: cost and radiation. It is certainly expensive. The radiation exposure is also a concern. Radiation exposure to humans comes mostly from cosmic radiation and radon. A significant amount now comes from X-rays and CT scans. Radiation exposure is cumulative. Long term exposure damages genetic material and increases the risk of cancer. No one knows the exact cutoff range. It is certainly prudent to avoid significant radiation exposure.

Abdominal CT scans can be extremely helpful in the diagnosis of acute appendicitis. Before CT was available, appendicitis was diagnosed clinically. Patients were often seen by a GS (general surgeon) and taken to the OR for exploratory surgery. We relied mostly on the patient history and exam. Cope's enlightening book *Early Diagnosis of the Acute Abdomen* (Ref. 2) was required reading. Even today, it remains an excellent resource. He highlighted the typical and many atypical presentations of appendicitis. In a typical case a patient would have a sudden onset of periumbilical pain, <u>followed</u> by nausea and vomiting. Later, the pain would migrate to the RLQ (Right Lower Quadrant) and localized tenderness would develop. Some cases had fever, many did not. About 2/3 cases had elevations in the WBC count, but this might occur late in the clinical course. Before the ready availability of abdominal CT scans these cases would have consultation with a GS. Many patients would be admitted to the hospital for observation or go directly to the OR for an "exploratory."

Nowadays the routine is to obtain a CT scan. One difficult decision for ER physicians is when to order a CT scan, especially in children. Most children with abdominal pain seen in the ER do not have appendicitis. Typically, the pain disappears on its own, likely cramping due to gas or constipation. Of course, CT scans shouldn't be used routinely unless appendicitis is quite likely. It would be time consuming, expensive and involve too much radiation exposure.

A frequent challenge for me would be handling the parents. Caring for Madeline was a typical case. Her concerned parents, Amy and Eric brought her in with abdominal pain. She was 5-years-old. That morning, Madeline awoke with some abdominal pain, wouldn't eat breakfast, and vomited twice. "She is lethargic. She's vomited before, but always seemed to improve quickly, and she still won't eat. We're worried she might have appendicitis."

After obtaining the history, I carefully did the exam. Madeline looked tired but in no acute distress. The VS were normal. She was minimally pale. Her lips and mucous membranes slightly dry. Her bowel sounds were hyperactive (typically bowel sounds are hypoactive in appendicitis). The abdomen was soft with mild diffuse tenderness. There was no localized tenderness in the RLQ. "She looks ill and dehydrated. We can observe her and start an IV to obtain blood and give a bolus of fluid. We'll check the urine and give one dose of antiemetic."

"What about a CT scan?" they asked.

"Better hold off for a bit. I don't think appendicitis is likely, and it's a lot of radiation for young children," I answered.

About an hour later the tests returned and I went back to evaluate the child. Madeline was improved. She was perky now; her slight pallor was gone. Repeat abdominal palpation showed no tenderness. "All of her blood and urine tests are normal." The nurses had given her a popsicle.

The parents however, remained skeptical. "Normal? What caused the abdominal pain and vomiting?" they asked.

"Usually, a virus or minor food poisoning. We can't be sure," I replied. This information didn't reassure them.

"We read that you need a CT scan to "Rule out" appendicitis. We want to be sure," they persisted.

I gave a long explanation about appendicitis, and how they can carefully and safely observe the child at home. Eric and Amy were not convinced.

I said, "Let's try this. Madeline: stand up here (she gets out of bed and stands). Follow me. Stand on one leg (we both stand on one leg), stand on the other leg (we both change legs). Now hop up and down (we're both hopping), the other leg (she follows)." I start hopping all around the room. Madeline smiling and laughing is hopping and chasing me. "We've been shaking her whole abdomen around, including her appendix. This can't be appendicitis," I explain. Amy and Eric nod in agreement. "I'll print out some instructions. Please bring her back if you notice any problems."

Critical Procedures

"Dr. Thomson I need you in room 10," the urgency in the RN's voice was obvious. I went immediately. There were two RNs and a tech already in the room. They were putting a gown on Aaron (a 12-year-old boy) starting an IV and attaching oxygen and HR monitors. His mother was standing nearby.

"What happened?" I asked.

His mother said, "About three hours ago he suddenly got some chest pain on the left side. It wasn't too bad. I gave him some Tylenol. About 20 minutes ago the pain got worse so we came to the ER."

As I listened, I examined Aaron. He was anxious and pale, sitting upright, taking shallow breaths with little grunts. He was splinting with each breath, obvious pleuritic pain. The oxygen was 97 %, RR 30, and HR 112. There were good breath sounds on the right, but markedly decreased on the left. Percussion (finger tapping) on the chest wall sounded hollow on the left side. He had a large pneumothorax.

A pneumothorax occurs when air escapes from the lung inside the chest and the lung collapses. This fairly common condition can occur "spontaneously." Most often due to a bleb, a minor congenital defect of alveoli (tiny air sacs), making a larger air sac. The wall of the bleb can rupture from a cough or sneeze, allowing air to escape. The patient has mild to moderate pain. Patients are typically admitted for careful observation. A small pneumothorax usually resolves on its own. Larger ones need a thoracostomy (chest) tube. This tube drains the escaped air and allows the lung to expand. A real danger is if enough air escapes it can develop high pressure or tension. This is a critical condition and rapidly fatal. Fortunately, it is quite rare. Death is caused by cardiac shock. What happens is the developing high pressure is transmitted across the entire chest and compresses everything, not just the lungs. The veins returning blood to the heart have very low blood pressure, about 5 (blood pressure in arteries is about 120 / 80). These low-pressure veins are easily compressed from a tension pneumothorax. This blocks blood flow into the heart. Poor flow in leads to poor flow out. Cardiac shock occurs, cardiac arrest can follow in minutes.

I checked for JVD. There were none. Dilated neck veins are often (but not always) present if chest veins are being compressed. No tracheal shift either. It didn't appear to be a tension pneumothorax at this point. I was still concerned. Aaron's VS were not too bad, but his respiratory distress (anxious, pale, rapid breathing and pleuritic pain) bothered me. I stayed at the bedside. "Real quick, call for a portable chest X-ray. Run to the trauma room and get a thoracostomy tray. Bring the suture cart to the bedside." This took about one minute. I took additional history. There was no fall or trauma. He was completely healthy, no medical problems. Oxygen 96 %; HR 116. I explained about the pneumothorax.

"Mom, you'd better sit in the chair. Your son will need a chest tube." I asked the staff to get ready in case we couldn't wait for the X-ray.

I opened the chest tube tray, drew up some lidocaine (anesthetic) into a syringe. The staff kept Aaron upright, removed his gown and held his left arm up.

For the first time, Aaron spoke, "Am I going to die?"

"Not today," was my quick response.

I noticed the HR was now 120. He seemed more uncomfortable. No time for sterile drapes. I splashed betadine over the axilla and rapidly injected the local anesthetic near the 4th rib. The radiology technician arrived with the portable X-ray machine.

"Don't you want a film?" she asked. Oxygen dropped to 92 %, HR increased to 136.

"No time," I grabbed a scalpel. "He might be developing a tension pneumo."

I quickly made a deep "Stab" incision through the skin in the left axilla. I took a few seconds to palpate the upper edge of the fourth rib. I saw the scalpel shaking. Why was that? Oh, it was attached to my hand. My right hand was shaking. I never noticed that before, but it didn't matter. This boy might have a cardiac arrest soon. I pushed the scalpel straight into the chest. A large whoosh of air surged out, confirming a tension pneumothorax. He didn't moan; the anesthetic worked perfectly. In seconds the HR started to drop: 140, 136, 130, 124, 118, 112. The critical danger was over.

We draped sterile towels around the area. I put a thoracostomy (chest) tube through the incision and placed a few stitches to secure the tube and reapproximate the skin. A dressing was applied, the procedure was over. The portable chest X-ray confirmed good tube placement and excellent expansion of the lung. He was admitted and transferred upstairs. Following up, I heard that he was discharged three days later and doing well.

As I was dictating the patient's note one of the nurses stopped by to discuss the case.

She asked, "Why didn't you put the needle in for the tension pneumothorax?"

Needle drainage for possible tension pneumothorax was a recommended initial procedure. A long 14-gauge (large bore) needle would be inserted below the clavicle on the affected side of the chest. In theory, the air under tension would rush out through the needle. The nurse had probably seen it attempted a few times.

"You know, I've tried that quite a few times. It never seems to work. Often the needle that is supplied in the kit wouldn't have a stylet. Even when it did, I couldn't get any air out. I think the needle gets blocked easily by tissue. Besides, in this case by the time I realized it was a tension pneumothorax I already had the scalpel in my hand. So, I just stabbed him with it."

———————————

Dr. Ashley Carter, a second-year resident, and I went to check on a patient in room 1, Resuscitation. Another attending and resident were in the middle of a "Code." An elderly man was found down at home, EMS was called. They began resuscitation and brought him to our ER. Like most of our codes it was not going well for the patient. He didn't respond to EMS efforts and became flatline (no electrical cardiac activity) upon arrival. The chances of a successful outcome from flatline were almost zero. CPR was in progress, the patient was intubated, and additional rounds of medications were being administered through a large bore peripheral (in the arm) IV. I suspected they physicians were about to "call it" shortly.

Seeing there were two resident physicians, I asked, "How about central IV access?"

"That doesn't usually make any difference," was their reply. I agreed. One could argue that medications given directly into the central circulation might be more effective, but in this code situation it would not be likely to change the outcome.

I asked, "Have you ever placed an IO line?" They had not. I was a bit surprised. They had never even seen one placed. "Let's put one in."

After a brief explanation, Ashley used the IO drill and placed the needle into the patient's right tibia. I highlighted the importance of immediately flushing the needle with three ccs of fluid. The needle tip is in the bone marrow. IV fluid and medications flow much better after the needle is flushed with high pressure. Any medications given through the IO needle enters the central venous circulation within seconds. One last dose of epinephrine was given through the IO needle, CPR was continued. A couple of minutes later the patient was pronounced dead.

The residents asked, "Have you ever seen an IO line work?"

"Absolutely," I replied. They were skeptical. All the EM residents I had worked with were adept at US guided IV line placement. This explained why they never had to use an IO line. In the ER IV access is essential. Most of our serious and critical cases would not

184

improve without IV fluid and medications. When the IO drill became available (10 years previously) I enthusiastically learned how to use it. On the next 10 or 12 patient "Codes" (resuscitations) I started an IO line on many of them. The procedure takes one minute, the central venous access was beautiful.

The residents questioned the ethics of "Practicing" on a patient during a code. The patient of course being unresponsive could not give consent. It was an excellent question and should always be a consideration. I explained that I started the IO in the cases where I had wanted central venous access. Instead of my usual subclavian or femoral line I would use the IO drill.

"Did it ever make a difference?" they asked.

"Many times," I answered. They looked upon me as if I were an old man, telling stories that we're no longer relevant in today's technologically advanced era. I asked the residents, "What if your US machine broke down? Haven't you run into a situation where your US guided IV lines were nearly impossible to place?"

At the Novi ER we had four small children living nearby with horrible seizure disorders. They presented many times with status epilepticus. Often, we were unable to place an IV line peripherally (due to all the jerking tonic clonic activity and the scarred veins from previous IV lines). The nurses would attempt IV access for two minutes. If not successful I would place the IO line.

"How many times have you drilled through the bone?"

"Never." Although I admitted that in small infants it would be a common complication. I had only placed one IO line in a newborn. The drilling technique is straightforward, but certainly takes

185

dexterity and "feel" or "touch" to control the depth. That is why they needed to practice, many times. Then, when the crucial time comes (and perhaps a young child's life would be hanging in the balance) they would be ready. It happened to me.

————————

My partner Dr. Caitlyn Wilson appeared frustrated, almost distraught. She was usually imperturbable, no matter the emergency. She'd been caring for a 56-year-old critically ill patient with apparent sepsis. This relatively young patient wasn't responding to treatment as expected.

"What's up?" I asked.

"I'm sending her to the ICU, but I don't think she's going to make it. I think she is septic; antibiotics are on board, I'm ordering a fourth bolus of IV fluids. Her BP initially, but now she's crashing. She has so much respiratory distress I'm going to intubate her soon," she replied.

"Want me to have a look?" I asked. It was about 6:15 PM. I had just signed out to another physician, so my slate was clear.

"Would you? That'd be great," Caitlyn replied.

I grabbed the portable US machine and walked quickly down the hall to room 7. Anyone would recognize this patient was in serious trouble: anxious, pale, cold, and clammy. She had severe tachypnea and tachycardia: 48 and 170 respectively. BP was 80/40, severe hypotension. There were two nurses at the bedside. "Let's get her to resuscitation room 1," I said. Placing the US probe over the anterior chest wall, immediately, clearly visible on the screen was a large pericardial effusion. This is a fluid collection in the sac around the heart. In this case it was under enough tension to restrict the flow of blood from the veins into the heart. If not enough blood enters the heart, not enough blood gets pumped into the aorta, and the patient goes into shock. IV fluids can help, but often is a temporizing measure. The only effective treatment would be to remove the pericardial fluid (pericardiocentesis). We didn't have much time.

We ran the patient and cart down to resuscitation. Dr. Wilson joined us on the way. "There's pericardial tamponade," have you done pericardiocentesis?" I asked.

"Never," she replied.

"Me either." We entered Resuscitation Room 1. I asked the unit tech to, "Call Surgery, Anesthesia, the Intensivist and Cardiology STAT. I'll see if there's anyone in the hospital that has done this before. Caitlyn, you intubate."

The Respiratory therapist arrived and prepped for intubation. I opened the pericardiocentesis tray. The physicians called back. Surgery, anesthesia, and the Intensivist hadn't done pericardiocentesis either. Cardiology had and would come in but were 10 to 15 minutes away. This patient could be dead by then. Caitlyn performed the intubation. The heart rate and blood pressure did not improve.

I was 20 years out from medical school and had performed pericardiocentesis only a handful of times. The first two in trauma labs "pretending" there was pericardial fluid and going through the motions. The other few times as a last-ditch attempt during codes when patients were failing all resuscitation efforts. Those attempts were years ago, before the use of portable ultrasound. The actual pericardiocentesis technique is straightforward. The physician inserts a long, large bore needle attached to a large 50 cc syringe. Starting below the xiphoid process, the needle is inserted through the upper abdominal wall towards the heart. The goal is to enter the pericardial space containing the excess fluid and drain it into the syringe. With drainage of the pericardial fluid the pressure should decrease, and the impaired venous return to the heart resolves, thereby restoring good blood flow to the patient.

"Do you want to do the pericardiocentesis Caitlyn?" I asked.

"No, you go ahead."

"Ok, no worries," I tried to sound confident. I splashed betadine over the upper abdomen and inserted the long 14-gauge needle just below the rib cage. I had limited US experience (we'd just recently obtained the portable machine) and was self-taught. Placing the US probe on the chest and then the abdomen, I couldn't visualize the needle and abandoned US guidance. Advancing the needle seven cm (2 inches) I felt a slight loss of resistance. Pulling back the syringe plunger, clear amber fluid filled the barrel. Fantastic! I quickly detached the syringe, disposed of the fluid, and repeated, removing 50 cc's each time. After 100, 150, 200 cc's, I checked the patient and VS each time. No response! This was serious trouble. Once enough fluid was withdrawn, the patient should rapidly improve. I was getting plenty of fluid, but there was absolutely no improvement. I removed an additional 50 cc's, then 100 cc's. Still, no response.

As I was abandoning hope the cardiologist arrived. "We're up to 300 cc's removed, and the HR and BP are not improving," I explained. He briefly checked the patient, looked at the syringe in my hand, and calmly suggested advancing the needle another few centimeters. I did. I felt a significant "Pop." The syringe immediately filled with bloody fluid. "Did I enter the heart?" I asked.

"No, no," the cardiologist replied. "Pericardial effusions are commonly bloody."

I quickly withdrew 50 cc's bloody fluid, 100 cc's. At 150 cc's there was a sudden change. Within seconds the patient's BP rocketed to 180 / 80. The heart rate fell from 170 to 100, (probably mine as well). The patient was out of immediate danger.

The cardiologist took over and threaded a wire into the pericardial sac, then slid a catheter over the wire to allow for continuous drainage of pericardial fluid. The critical pericardial tamponade resolved. The now stable patient was transferred to the ICU. The now calm and collected emergency physician (me) went home.

––––––––––––––––––

A 38-year-old man presented to the ER on December 15th, two hours after a fight at a local tavern. He admitted to having a few drinks, was sitting at a table talking with friends, then suddenly was "Sucker" punched in the left eye. Initially he had moderate left eye pain, but it had gotten progressively worse and was now severe. He hadn't noticed any double vision; the swelling had closed his eyelids shut. He denied LOC, neck pain, malocclusion (change in bite), or other injuries. On exam his VS were stable, the GCS score 15, and he appeared uncomfortable due to the left eye pain. He smelled of alcohol but had no slurred speech or incoordination.

A brief trauma survey showed no injuries, except to the face. There was significant ecchymotic swelling over the left orbit, closing the eyelids together tightly. He had facial bony tenderness on the lower lateral portion of the left orbit. The teeth were intact and stable. The right pupil was normal size and reactive to light, the EOMs (eye movements) intact. He had good vision in the right eye. Using two retractors I was able to pry open the swollen left eyelids. There was significant hemorrhage (blood) in the left anterior chamber (front part of the eye). I could barely visualize the pupil, it appeared unreactive to light. He said he couldn't see anything with his left eye, couldn't count fingers, and couldn't even detect light. I looked carefully, comparing both eyes. I wasn't sure but thought there was proptosis (displacement forward) of the left eye. "There is serious bleeding in, and I suspect behind your left eye. Obviously, you've lost vision on that side. We'll send you for a STAT CT scan."

A traumatic injury causing complete loss of vision is fortunately quite rare. One of the few reversible causes is a retrobulbar hematoma (bleeding behind the eyeball). This can compress the optic nerve and cause visual loss in the affected eye. Depending on the amount of blood and pressure on the optic nerve the decreased vision can quickly become permanent. The optic nerve is well protected by the bony skull, but it is easily damaged by pressure (unlike peripheral nerves which are tough and not easily damaged). If diagnosed early and the blood removed quickly, occasionally vision can be improved or restored. The procedure is a lateral canthotomy. The practitioner cuts through the lateral (outside) portion of tissue next to the eye, then probes with a hemostat behind the eyeball. The hematoma (blood) is drained and pressure on the optic nerve is relieved. It takes a few minutes.

I placed the order for a STAT CT scan of the left orbit. I called the CT techs, "He should be the next patient on the table. Let the radiologist know that I need an immediate report. Thanks." I asked Jo Anne, the unit clerk to contact the ophthalmologist on call, the senior surgical resident as well as the in-house trauma surgeon (we had recently been certified as a Level 1 Trauma Center). I found Dr. George Fisher, my emergency physician partner working with me that evening, and asked, "Have you ever performed or seen a lateral canthotomy?"

"No," he replied. This procedure was rare, and even more rare to be performed by an ER physician. I had 60 partners in my group. I had never heard of any of us performing a lateral canthotomy.

It had been years since I'd read about the procedure. "Can you bring up a video on our computer?" George started typing.

The calls came back. The senior surgical resident and trauma surgeon both had not done the procedure and said they wouldn't be any help. Dr. Jones, the on-call eye specialist said he was only covering the first two weeks of the month. I asked the unit tech to call the next ophthalmologist and walked around the corner to the CT scanner control room.

There were two CT techs who were just starting to bring the images up on their computer. "Uh oh, that looks like a large hematoma behind the left eye. Doesn't it?" I asked.

"It has to be," they answered.

I called the radiologist, "What do you think?"

"There is a large retrobulbar hematoma. Likely from a fracture of the inferior and lateral orbital bones," he answered. I walked quickly back to the ER.

Dr. Fisher had found a video of the procedure. We reviewed it together. "Looks like I'll have to do the lateral canthotomy. Do you want to help?"

"Not really," he said. That surprised me.

"At least you'd be seeing one for the first time," I mentioned.

"I'll try to step in," he replied without enthusiasm. George went to see his own patients.

I went to the patient's room. Brenda brought in the "Plastics Tray" (a complete wound care kit with sterile equipment. I was happy to see her. She was the head ER technician, and in charge of stocking supplies. She knew where every piece of equipment was in the entire department. Better yet, Brenda was imperturbable. No matter the chaos, she was always calm. Frequently she would be handing me an instrument before I had even asked. She drove her coworkers crazy with her compulsiveness (a small price to pay for her dedication and expertise).

My portable phone rang. "Dr. Johnson, hello. This is Mark Thomson in the ER. I need to do a lateral canthotomy….."

"Stop right there. I'm not on call. Dr. Jones is covering Ophthalmology," he interrupted.

"I just spoke with Dr. Jones. He said he was on call the first two weeks of December," I explained.

"That's incorrect," Dr. Johnson said angrily. "He's on call for the first half of the month. I start tomorrow, the 16th."

"I see; but it's 11:40 PM, would you stay on the line for a few minutes and talk me through the procedure?"

"No. You have to contact Dr. Jones," he said emphatically.

I hung up. The patient was returning from CT. There wasn't any more time.

"The CT scan shows a large hematoma behind your left eye. It's a collection of blood. I need to make an incision on the side of your eye and try to remove it." The patient agreed.

Brenda had the tray opened; the equipment ready. I washed my hands and donned sterile gloves. Using 1 % lidocaine with epinephrine I injected the lateral canthus (tissue next to his left eye). Using a hemostat, I compressed the area for about a minute, to minimize bleeding. Using scissors, I made a two cm incision. With forceps to retract the lateral portion of the lower lid downward the lateral canthal ligament was exposed. I cut through this ligament with scissors. Taking a small, curved hemostat I dissected toward the retrobulbar area. Suddenly, about 15 cc's (one tablespoon) of dark blood with small clots drained out. Pretty straightforward. The operation took four minutes. The patient tolerated the procedure well, having minimal discomfort.

I had a bit of hope that over time some of his vision might return. A week later I spoke with his ophthalmologist. The patient could see light but did not regain any useful vision.

Young Partners

One morning in Jackson, I was about to intubate a patient using our recently acquired fiberoptic laryngoscope. This scope with advanced technology was a fantastic piece of equipment. It allowed a beautiful view of the vocal cords during intubation, even for difficult patients (morbidly obese, vomiting, bleeding, etc). The goal of intubation is to secure the airway by placing a breathing tube safely through the vocal cords and into the proximal trachea. Just before starting the RSI I asked a tech to find Dr. Davis and ask him to come over. I'd been able to use the fiberoptic scope about 10 times and wanted to share my experience with him and possibly compare notes.

Dr. Caleb Davis was a young residency trained emergency medicine physician with a great enthusiastic attitude. He came into the room, "Hey Caleb, I'm going to use the fiberoptic scope. Do you have much experience with it?"

"Oh yes, quite a bit," he replied. "We were able to use it during our third year."

A minute or two later, after giving sedative and paralytic medications, I inserted the fiberoptic laryngoscope with my left hand, and easily visualized the vocal cords. Grasping the ET tube with my right hand I advanced it towards the cords. This time (and on a previous attempt about a week before) I couldn't quite get the tip anteriorly enough to pass it through the vocal cords. After about 20 seconds, I removed the ET tube to allow bag mask ventilation with 100 % oxygen to avoid hypoxia.

Before the fiberoptic scope physicians used a solid metal laryngoscope. We would insert a malleable stylet inside the ET tube and would bend the stylet tip anteriorly. This would bend the ET tube tip anteriorly and allow passage of the ET tube through the cords. A curved rigid stylet was supplied for use inside the ET tube when using the fiberoptic scope.

The RT was bagging and ventilating the sedated and paralyzed patient. Caleb spoke up, "Dr. Thomson I noticed you were holding the ET tube in the middle. Try holding by the black stylet handle (on the proximal end). You should be able to control the tube tip." On my second attempt I again readily visualized the vocal cords. The ET tube tip was still a bit posterior to the vocal cords. I couldn't safely advance it. Holding the stylet by the black handle, I lifted my wrist a bit. The tip of the ET tube immediately moved anteriorly, pointing perfectly through the open vocal cords. I advanced the ET tube over the stylet and directly through the vocal cords. Voila! The patient's trachea was safely intubated, the airway secured.

"That was great Caleb, thanks." The assembled team, respiratory therapist, two RNs, and two techs could see my talented partner was as comfortable with airway management as the "Senior" physician with over 30 years' experience. They must have been as impressed as I was. It wasn't the first time I thought I might be teaching one of my younger partners and it turned out that I was the one receiving the lesson.

One extremely challenging scenario for any physician is a newborn with fever. The differential diagnosis is long and includes many life-threatening illnesses. Complications from pregnancy and labor need to be considered. Signs and symptoms (that often guide patient management decisions) are typically subtle or absent in the neonate. All newborn infants are small, about seven lbs. IVs and procedures can be extremely difficult, even for experienced providers, in tiny wiggling patients. Infections are top on the list of likely possibilities. The immune system of neonates is not well developed, they do not have much reserve. They can become hypoxic and acidotic quickly and become critically ill. Treatment of infections early in their course can avoid death and serious disability.

I had just arrived for my shift; the ER was hopping. The electronic chart list had 24 patients waiting to be seen. We had resident physicians working alongside each of us. They can be a huge help, especially in their second and third year. Dr. Paul Mann, a second-year emergency medicine resident, was assigned to me. We clicked on the first patient: A three day old with a fever. VS: temperature of 101.2 degrees, RR 48, HR 180. No question there was a documented fever. The cutoff for normal was 100.4. I asked Paul to start the history and exam. This newborn would need a full sepsis workup: IV, blood tests and cultures, bladder catheterization for urine tests and culture, chest X-ray and a LP. I went to the charge RN Kathy. She assigns the ER staff throughout the department.

"We need two nurses, a tech, and an LP tray in room 17. There's a newborn with a fever who needs a full septic workup."

"We're swamped, but we'll manage somehow," she replied.

I went to the bedside, "What's the story Paul?"

He presented the case. "This is a 3-day-old boy, born vaginally at 39 weeks gestation without pre or perinatal complications. He breastfed well the first two days, but not since midnight. He is irritable and has been crying nonstop. The mother noticed he felt warm this morning, called the pediatrician, and was referred to the ER. He has no vomiting or diarrhea, no jaundice."

"How about your exam?" I asked.

"I couldn't find any source for the fever."

I examined the child. He was irritable with a persistent, but normal sounding and strong cry. There was mild acrocyanosis (purplish discoloration on the hands and feet, a normal finding in a newborn). The anterior fontanelle wasn't bulging. He had good breath sounds on chest auscultations, and the femoral pulses were strong. There was no rash, jaundice, or hepatosplenomegaly.

"What's the plan, Paul? I asked.

"Septic workup and LP."

"Absolutely," I responded. "You put in all the orders. Include a portable chest X-ray. Order the antibiotics now, so they can be started immediately after we do the LP. What should we start?"

"Ampicillin and gentamicin?" Paul replied.

"Perfect." I explained to the mother, "We need blood, urine, and spinal fluid. Infants with a fever can easily have serious infections that are hard to find. To get the spinal fluid we need to do a

Lumbar Puncture. The resident and I will put a thin needle in the lower back. We'll try to obtain about a teaspoon of spinal fluid. This will be examined under the microscope and cultured for infection. He'll be started on antibiotics and then admitted to the hospital." The nursing staff was preparing to start the IV. "We definitely need blood cultures," I said, double checking. "After the IV, straight cath the bladder for urine analysis and culture."

I opened the LP kit, while the nurses obtained the urine sample. "We'll do the spinal tap together. You can have the first attempt." Paul and I each palpated the space between lumbar 3 and 4. The spinal cord ends at L1, so inserting a needle into the spinal cord at the L3 / L4 interspace is safe. I marked the correct interspace with a marking pen. One assistant gently restrained the child, another watched the oxygen and heart rate monitors. Paul used a short 25-gauge spinal needle and advanced the tip slowly 1 to 2 cm (half an inch). Upon removing the stylet there was a return of clear spinal fluid. It seemed to drip quickly, perhaps the spinal fluid pressure was increased. This could indicate meningitis. We put one cc of fluid into each of four sterile tubes and placed a Band-Aid over the puncture site. The child settled down, there was less crying. That made meningitis more likely. The LP, by removing fluid, can relieves a little spinal pressure.

We went to our workstation to finish entering orders and page the pediatric hospitalist for admission. "Add a bolus of normal saline and the antiviral acyclovir. Order CSF (cerebrospinal fluid) bacterial and viral cultures, and a PCR (polymerase chain reaction test) for Herpes virus. Then go check and make sure the antibiotics have been started," I instructed.

"The ampicillin is hanging, and the gentamycin is at the bedside," Paul said.

I checked the clock and the patient's registration time. Right about 50 minutes after arrival. Wow, that was fantastic. About the quickest septic work up and spinal tap on an infant that I'd ever been involved in. The triage RN had recognized the potential for serious illness and marked the infant's chart as a level V, putting it to the top of the patients to be seen list. I complimented Paul and the staff, thanking them for their excellent performance. The IV, urine cath, and LP procedures were all done smoothly on their first attempts.

Shortly, the initial test results returned. The blood tests were unremarkable, the urine clear, the chest X-ray negative.

We discussed the case with the pediatrician for admission. He reviewed our antibiotic choice, "Good."

"I also started acyclovir," I mentioned. Covering newborn patients with sepsis of unknown etiology for a Herpes infection had recently been under discussion in the medical literature. It was not yet standard practice.

"Oh, ok. Probably a good idea," he replied quizzically. "Did the mother have a Herpes infection?"

"No, and the child doesn't have a rash. I thought it best though to cover all the bases." Often the mother and obstetrician are unaware of herpes infections in the birth canal. They can be asymptomatic and difficult to diagnose. The spinal fluid results returned. The protein level was increased, and there were 40 WBC's (white blood cells) per high power field. Half were lymphocytes. This indicated meningitis, a very dangerous infection around the brain, especially for newborns. On the repeat exam the child appeared stable. It was wait and see how this infant would respond over the next few days. He was transferred to the neonatal unit on the pediatric floor.

Five days later I bumped into the same pediatrician. He was in the ER, admitting another patient. "How's that newborn doing, the one with meningitis?" I asked.

"Great. You won't believe it!" he exclaimed. "The PCR was positive. He was diagnosed with Herpes meningitis, and the viral culture confirmed it."

"How's he doing?" I repeated.

"Beautifully, no complications at all. The child developed a mild viral exanthem (rash). He responded to the acyclovir and will probably be discharged in another few days."

"That's fantastic!" I replied. What a tremendous outcome. By starting the antiviral medication in the ER, we likely saved the newborn's life and prevented serious lifelong neurologic disability, seizures, and mental deficiency. I thought for a moment, then became a bit upset. "Hey," I irritatedly asked the Pediatrician. "Did anyone think to call us back?" (About our care and treatment of this baby in the ER. Nearly all the calls we would get back from the admitting doctors were complaints, usually regarding minor issues).

The pediatrician paused, then apologized. They had been using this as a teaching case. This was a rare infection and up to this time most of the cases anyone had been involved with had poor outcomes. "You're right. We should have called. Thank you."

I circled around the ER and found the staff who'd cared for this infant. I let them know that their skill and efforts were responsible for the wonderful outcome and saving the baby's life. Most of the time, when we dramatically intervene to prevent death, it involves elderly patients. Unfortunately, many of those patients will soon succumb to their serious underlying disease. In this case a newborn, its whole life ahead of him, will be normal. The best "Save" I was ever involved in, and no one had noticed.

"Can you find Dr. Gilbert and ask her to step in for a moment?" I asked the tech. I was in the middle of placing a thoracostomy (chest)tube. The patient had come in via EMS with complaints of chest pain and shortness of breath. He was transferred from the EMS cart onto a special Big Boyz Bariatric Bed. He was the biggest patient I had ever treated. Weighing a staggering 612 lbs. On exam his breath sounds were diminished bilaterally due to his morbid obesity and massively thick chest wall, but even more so on the left side. A portable chest X-ray confirmed a pneumothorax of about 50 % on that side. He would need a chest tube. I asked surgery if they were available to perform the procedure (which I knew would be challenging). They said, "Not for a while. We're busy with two trauma patients."

Placing thoracostomy tubes is usually a straightforward procedure. The physician palpates the third and fourth rib area in the patient's axilla. It is an area known as the "Zone of Safety" because of the lack of any important structures near that location. After prepping the skin and injecting a local anesthetic, an incision is made with a scalpel. A long, curved hemostat is used to bluntly dissect (divide) the tissue down to the ribs. Then the instrument is carefully pushed over the top of the rib (there is an artery, vein, and nerve along the bottom of each rib) and pushed through the pleura (lining of the lung). A chest tube is passed through this opening and sutured into place. The tube is connected to a small amount of negative pressure to remove air or fluid.

There were two ER techs assisting me. I had bluntly dissected towards the ribs but was now stymied. This massively obese individual had at least 12 to 14 inches of fatty tissue in his left axilla. I had lengthened my initial incision to allow room to dissect deeper. I was buried up to my wrists and still couldn't palpate the patient's ribs. I was using a headlamp, but visibility deep in the hole of tissue was limited.

Dr. Karyn Gilbert arrived. "What's up Mark?" she inquired.

I was happy to see her. Karyn was another of my young physician partners. She had great clinical knowledge and procedural skills. Her demeanor was unique. She thought that at any moment a disaster was about to happen (in this busy ER she was often right). She also possessed a fantastic dry sense of humor which she did not hesitate to use. This was badly needed on our tough days. I enjoyed working alongside her.

"Karyn, it's good to see you. I'm struggling here. There is so much adipose tissue in his axilla that I can't find and palpate his ribs. Any suggestions?"

She took a moment, looked at my large incision, peered briefly into the depth of the dissection, then shook her head in the negative. "Nope. Dig deeper." She left to attend to her own patients. Wow. That didn't seem like much help.

I took the longest thoracic clamp we had and dug down another two inches. This time I was able to palpate a rib. I wasn't sure if it was number 3, 4, or 5. I pushed the clamp over the top edge and felt a "pop" as I broke through the pleura and into the chest cavity. Fantastic! I finished placing the chest tube quickly. Good position was confirmed by a portable chest X-ray. The patient tolerated the procedure well (without complications). I went to find Dr. Gilbert. She was at the workstation with another attending, two residents and a few scribes and nurses.

"Thanks for nothing Dr. Gilbert," I hollered with as much anger as I could muster. "I asked for your help, and you abandoned me in my time of need!"

Karyn was stunned, mouth agape. The room fell silent. I paused as long as I was able, then burst into laughter. I explained that upon hearing her advice of "Dig Deeper" I thought "Thanks for nothing." But after a moment I realized it was perfect advice. I dug deeper and was immediately successful. For once, I was able to catch Dr. Gilbert off guard.

Vaccines

He was 4-years-old and he was dying. Two days before coming to the ER, he was seen by his pediatrician and diagnosed with an ear infection. He was placed on an oral antibiotic. He seemed unchanged until the night before when he developed a fever which responded to Tylenol. The next morning, he awoke with a high fever, was delirious, and had a bad rash. The parents brought him directly to our ER. The child's history was unremarkable, except the parents did not have him immunized. The child was critically ill. He was hypotensive (low BP), his neck was stiff, and there was a diffuse maculopapular (splotchy) rash with red and purplish blotches. His hands and feet were cyanotic from poor perfusion. We did the septic work up, started oxygen, IV fluids and antibiotics, and called the Pediatric Critical Care EMS unit for transfer. His BP improved a bit and the cyanosis resolved, but I was not optimistic.

The pediatric intensivist asked why I hadn't done the spinal tap. I told him that at this point the child was too unstable, when we rolled him onto his side the cyanosis worsened. There were case reports of unstable, seriously ill children having a cardiac or respiratory arrest when positioning them for a lumbar puncture. I explained to the parents their child likely had meningitis and was critically ill. We hoped for the antibiotics to take effect.

The next day I called the Pediatric ICU. The child had stable VS for four to six hours. They were able to perform the LP. Shortly thereafter he went into septic shock. They administered two vasopressors simultaneously but couldn't keep the child's BP up. Blood and spinal fluid tests revealed H inf (Haemophilus). The young child died 16 hours after transfer. In the 1990's an effective vaccine for H inf bacteria was developed. Immediately the three or four dose regimens became part of the routine pediatric vaccination schedule. The incidence of serious H inf bacterial infection (pneumonia and meningitis) decreased markedly. This was the only H inf meningitis case I saw after the vaccine came out. Knowing that it was easily preventable made the tragedy even worse.

Similarly, over my first 20 years of practice I saw five or six cases of meningitis due to Pneumococcus. In 2002 the Pneumococcal vaccine became widely available. It was quickly adopted into the routine pediatric vaccine schedule. The vaccine was fantastically effective. I saw only one case of pneumococcal meningitis during the last 16 years of my career. It was in an unimmunized child. That child also died. It wasn't only my experience. Pneumococcal meningitis became rare in vaccinated individuals. One or two pokes in the arm would have prevented another tragedy.

———————————

It is difficult for me to understand the controversy about vaccinations. Doubts about vaccines are nothing new and have been around since the late 1700's (when inoculations were first developed). When the topic of vaccinations came up, I'd recommend people read one of the many articles about Dr. Edward Jenner and the history of smallpox and vaccination (Ref. 3).

In childhood I witnessed the tremendous decrease in serious infections when effective vaccines become available. Around 1960 I remember seeing two victims of polio. They lived in the small town of Chelsea. One had a limp withered and paralyzed left arm, the other braces on both nearly useless legs. Parents were terrified of this silent, unseen polio virus, striking without warning. It could cause death or permanent disability, often in perfectly healthy young people. I have a clear recollection of when the polio vaccine came to town. Every kindergartner was lined up in the gymnasium at South Street Elementary School, getting poked in the arm. Polio disappeared in a few years, nearly eradicated worldwide.

Vaccines are among the safest of all medical interventions. Serious complications from vaccines are exceedingly rare. I have been at the bedside caring for children and adults, dying from vaccine preventable infections. I have spoken to their heartbroken families. I don't tell them the tragedy was easily avoidable, by a couple pokes in the arm. It's too late. There is no reason to add to their inconsolable grief. I am not sure I can convince anyone who is against vaccination to change their mind. I am convinced they have not been at the bedside; they have not seen what I have seen.

I was always concerned about new infectious diseases, especially viruses. Ebola, SARS (severe acute respiratory syndrome), MERS (middle eastern respiratory syndrome), Zika, West Nile, etc. With 7.8 billion people on the planet the incidence of severe contagious disease increases. Many of these infections can be transmitted to healthcare providers, some with high fatality rates (over 30 percent). New viral pathogens are always emerging.

For ten years, I was chair of the hospital Ethics Committee. We discussed policies and procedures to adopt if and when severe infectious diseases presented to our facility. I asked what we should do about employee absenteeism? The other committee members weren't concerned. "Our workers were dedicated." I pointed out that in 2004 during the SARS outbreak in Toronto health care providers not showing up for their shift had become a problem. About 25 percent of nurses caring for SARS patients caught the infection. Almost 10 percent of those nurses died! I was outvoted, "Any employee not arriving for their shift would be terminated." I thought that was harsh. I considered myself a dedicated health care worker, but coming in to care for patients knowing that about 10 percent of us could die? I wasn't sure what I would do. Many physicians, nurses and staff working in the ER had young children. My children were grown. I hoped I'd have the courage to continue working, so they could stay home and protect their families. A few months passed. I was somewhat relieved when I wasn't asked to continue my volunteer assignment on the ethics committee.

A similar issue arose with Covid. Any employee who could be immunized but refused vaccination would be terminated. Pretty harsh. I hoped they would get vaccinated.

It was October in 2014 when a mother brought her son Nathan, 10-years-old to the ER. "His right hand is weak," she said emphatically. New onset unilateral extremity weakness is rare in children. I was immediately concerned. In 30 years, I'd only seen two cases. One was caused by a brain tumor, the other by a stroke. Sixty years ago, the common cause was polio. This child's weakness started three days prior, she noticed him having trouble using utensils to eat. They went to the pediatrician's office the day before. The doctor couldn't document any weakness.

Nathan looked perfectly healthy. His only other symptom was aching in the right arm. His history was negative. I carefully performed a complete neurological exam. I couldn't find any weakness until I checked for an arm drift. I had Nathan close his eyes and hold both hands out in front with the palms up. There was minimal lowering of the right arm, and the wrist pronated (turned inward). The mother was correct, there was definite mild weakness. I assured her that we would do a thorough investigation. Nathan's blood work returned normal. His CT scan showed no tumor or stroke. The pediatrician was hesitant to admit the child, not believing I found mild weakness. I insisted. There had been recent case reports of unexplained extremity weakness and paralysis in children.

A few weeks later the pediatrician asked if I'd heard about Nathan. She informed me that he was diagnosed with AFM (Acute Flaccid Myelitis) and developed paralysis of his right arm, likely permanent. AFM is an inflammatory reaction in the spinal cord following a minor upper respiratory tract infection. It is similar to Polio but may be due to an enterovirus (EV-D68 or EV-A71). There are no effective treatments. Fortunately, AFM has remained rare. If it becomes common, the best hope may be a vaccine.

Lacerations

Halfway through my career our physician group began to employ MLPs (mid-level providers), NPs (nurse practitioners) and PAs (physician assistants). This development was a national trend. Most MLPs have four years of college followed by four years of postgraduate education. I found them to be dedicated and enthusiastic. They worked closely alongside us throughout the ER. After a year or so of clinical experience they would routinely provide excellent emergency care and treatment. They took over laceration repair. Stitching lacerations was straightforward but somewhat time consuming.

I was hesitant to give up the procedures. Wound care was relaxing. Taking 10 to 20 minutes, sitting quietly at the bedside, and listening to patient stories was enjoyable, and provided a break from the chaotic ER environment. Many of the best anecdotes were from elderly patients. They were good story tellers, perhaps because they lived before visual television replaced auditory radio. To "Age" has developed a bad reputation. One definition of aging is: to sit quietly and acquire a desired characteristic. While I would be suturing, many seniors were eager to share a bit of their acquired wisdom and life history.

———————————

Mr. Emerson was in his early 90s, walking slowly and carefully to the exam room. He came in due to a laceration on his left leg, from the edge of a bucket. He had brushed against it in his garage. After exploring the wound and starting my repair I asked him, "You wouldn't be related to the Emerson Orchard family, would you?" Emerson's Orchard was a popular destination in the fall for many families, especially those with young children (including mine).

"Oh yes. My father started the orchard about 75 years ago. It's been in the family ever since," he stated with pride.

"Are you still running the place?" I asked, already knowing the answer.

"Not anymore. My son and now his children have taken over."

In 2003 our family bought an old run-down farm. I cleared brush from 16 acres and planted hay. I tried growing paw trees, but they grew slowly, and pollination was sporadic. After seven years the fall harvest was a paltry 50 100 papaws. I asked Mr. Emerson what it was like running an orchard. It seemed like a thriving, successful business.

He said it had been a long road. A lot of struggles and hard times, especially in the early days. They had tried all kinds of fruit: apples, pears, cherries, and peaches. Not many people were interested in pears. The cherry and peaches were hard to maintain and get good crops. Often, late spring frosts would spoil pollination. They always relied on apples. With the different varieties, better equipment and spraying patterns a good crop and harvest could be counted on. "I have great grandchildren running around the orchard now," he said contentedly.

"Dr. Thomson, it's your brother calling." That was unusual. I had five brothers, two lived close by. They rarely called when I was working. I went to the office. On the line was Dan, obviously concerned, "Becky fell and cut her forehead on the fireplace hearth. It's BAD." Becky was his rambunctious three-year-old daughter. Young children fall and sustain lacerations to the head and face frequently. The wound often spurts blood dramatically due to the highly vascular tissue. Beyond a minor scar there is seldom significant damage. I was relieved it was likely nothing serious.

I asked Dan, "How big is the cut?"

"BIG," he replied, his voice nervous with anxiety.

"How long is it?" I asked.

"SIX INCHES!"

Wow. A six-inch laceration across the forehead of a 3-year-old. That would be big. "Go measure it with a ruler."

He returned to the phone a minute later, "It's one inch long."

I told him to press some gauze over the cut and bring her to the ER. Hanging up the phone I had to smile. Dan was two years younger than I, and a tremendous athlete. Lightning fast with excellent coordination he became a fantastic tennis player. We marveled at his always calm demeanor. "Ice water in his veins," certainly applied to him. Until this episode I couldn't recall ever seeing him upset. Discovering a bleeding facial laceration on his darling daughter had done it. Underneath his imperturbable exterior, he had the same emotions as the rest of his brothers. Dan and Becky arrived a few minutes later. The laceration was easily repaired.

I wouldn't get off so easily the next time. A few months later Becky somehow cut her tongue deeply. This was before the time of using sedation in the ER. With two assistants and bedsheet wrapping for restraint we wrestled around with her for quite some time. I was able to pry her mouth open and place a few large absorbable sutures. The key was putting the first one in the tip of the tongue. With vigorous traction it was possible to pull the tongue forward enough to enable placement of additional sutures. That was over 30 years ago. Her scars are invisible today.

Working in Jackson one evening, Mrs. Little came in. I grew up in Chelsea, a small town nearby. The name was familiar, there was a Mrs. Little on my paper route. That was 48 years ago. This Mrs. Little was 85-years-old, on blood thinners (warfarin), and had slipped and fallen while shoveling snow from her walk. I didn't recognize her. I checked the address: 637 Madison Street. That was the house, she had to be the lady on my paper route. She didn't recognize me.

I chided her for shoveling snow. "You should hire a high school kid to do it."

"There was only an inch," she replied. There was an ugly bruise on the side of her forehead, but she was neurologically intact. Her blood work returned just fine, including the INR (a measurement of blood thinner amount). A CT scan of her head was normal, there was no bleeding. I admitted her to the observation unit overnight, for repeated neurologic checks.

I hesitated to tell her that I was her paperboy many years ago. It was my first job. I told my parents, "I want a bike, just like my friend's."

"You can buy a bike. Get a paper route," was their reply. I think the bike cost $16.95.

What I recalled about Mrs. Little was that she was a pleasant lady, but somewhat unhappy with my delivery service. Most days I would fold the papers and instead of walking all the way to the porch I would try a long throw from the front sidewalk. I missed the porch a few times. That was 50 years ago. I wondered what she might think about having a paperboy (who couldn't deliver the paper correctly) now be her doctor. I didn't mention it.

———————————

Mr. McKernan was 65-years-old and came to the ER with a cut on his left hand. He dropped his coffee cup and tried to catch it before it hit the table. I injected the wound with a local anesthetic, looked carefully for any foreign body, and began to reapproximate the wound edges with sutures.

"What do you do for a living?" I asked.

He was just about to retire. He had started out as an auto mechanic, working for many years in the back of an automobile dealership. Eventually he became the manager of the repair department. We realized that diagnosing a car problem was similar to diagnosing a medical problem. You take a history of the complaints (symptoms), examine the engine (signs), perhaps run a few tests, and diagnose the trouble. In the 100-year history of cars he pointed out the basics hadn't changed: engine, drive shaft, steering, brakes, wheels, tires.

I was bandaging his wound when he said, "Let me ask you something." This was the second time when his hand suddenly became numb. This time it felt weak and uncoordinated. Wow, this new information was concerning. I hadn't asked about why he had dropped the coffee cup. I asked more questions, did an exam for a possible stroke. He was admitted for a likely TIA (transient ischemic attack / mini stroke). I later found out he had a cardiac echo bubble study positive for a PFO (Patent Foramen Ovale, a small hole between the two upper heart chambers). He underwent a catheterization procedure to close the hole in his heart. This likely prevented a future stroke. What good fortune that he had spoken up.

In 2016, I was working in Jackson, it was wintertime, and the department was swamped. Our "Fast track" area was overwhelmed. They placed Mr. Nieminen, a 93-year-old man into the main ER. "I'm Dr. Thomson, what happened?" He was with his daughter. He'd been trimming a board with a bandsaw to make a smaller piece for whittling. The tip of his right thumb was nearly amputated. "An old man with power tools," was the mantra for severe hand injuries. I cautioned him about using tools.

The daughter spoke up emphatically, "You can be sure about that."

I could see who was in charge. The elderly gentleman wasn't looking very happy. I explored the wound. There was some bone exposed, but no serious injury. With 8 to 10 sutures, we could likely save all the injured tissue.

When Mr. Nieminen spoke, I recognized a heavy Finnish accent. "Are you from around here? I inquired.

"Oh no. I just moved down here a couple of months ago. My wife died last year, and my daughter wants to keep an eye on me," he reported.

"You're from the UP?" I asked. "My parents were born and raised in the Upper Peninsula of Michigan."

"You bet. I lived in Calumet all my life."

"Calumet," I exclaimed, "Your whole life? You must have known my great uncle. He's dead now. He lived in Calumet. His name was Leo Lucchesi."

Mr. Nieminen gazed off into the distance reflecting and said, "Leo Lucchesi. I knew Leo Lucchesi."

"Oh, you're pulling my leg," I teased.

He said, "I remember going to the county fairgrounds in the 1930's. I was 12-years-old, and Leo Lucchesi had an airplane. He was taking off and landing, first time I ever saw an airplane. I'll never forget it."

I finished suturing and went to print out the discharge information. When I returned his daughter showed me a picture (on her cell phone, which she found on the internet) from The Calumet News. It was my great uncle, leaning against an airplane. The caption read Leo Lucchesi, Calumet County. The world was a smaller place back in the 1930's. For a few minutes in a busy ER in 2018 it was smaller again.

A 24-year-old woman and her mother were in room 12. The young woman was hesitant and anxious. She had a small bleeding laceration on her left index finger. Putting gauze and pressure over the cut the bleeding was easily controlled.

"How did that happen?" I asked.

"I was cutting a bagel," she replied.

"You are right-handed." I stated.

"Yes," she answered, "How did you know?"

"The left hand always gets hurt. People hold a knife with their dominant hand. Are you from Germany?" I inquired, thinking I heard a German accent.

"Oh no. We're French."

I was puzzled for a moment, then guessed, "From Alsace-Lorraine (a cultural region in eastern France on the west bank of the Rhine River next to Germany)?"

They started laughing and smiling. "Yes! How did you know that?"

"I have a twin brother, Michael. On foreign study in college, he was living in Strasbourg. When I was able to visit him, I noticed the people around there spoke with a mixture of French and German. He told me about Alsace-Lorraine."

The laceration was easily repaired, and off went my new friends.

———————————

An 88-year-old farmer was driven to the ER by his wife after cutting his left palm deeply with a knife. He was initially seen by a PA but sent to my area for possible flexor tendon injuries.

"How'd this happen?" I asked.

"I went out to the barn and did a few chores. I used my pocketknife to cut some twine, missed and got a little cut," he told me matter of factly. A "little" cut on the hand didn't seem to concern him. Upon examination this man had significant arthritis in all the joints of his hands, and a small tremor, likely familial. There was a long, deep cut across the entire left palm. I could see four flexor tendons. I had him slowly flex and extend all his fingers, carefully inspecting each tendon throughout this range of motion. The tendons were intact, no injury at all. That was lucky! Flexor tendon injuries usually required closure in the OR, and carried quite a risk of scarring, decreased range of motion and disability.

"This is a large laceration. We'll wash it thoroughly to decrease the risk of infection. We'll patch you up in no time."

I knew about cutting twine. My children help me bale hay on our own farm. There is no better feeling of contentment than to stand in an old dirt floor hay barn after a long day of baling. Late in the evening the breeze lays down, the light fades, and you can rest and enjoy the sweet smell of fresh hay.

I asked the old man, "Do you have hay in your barn?" Turns out he and his wife had lived in their house on a 100-acre farm for about 70 years. They always produced hay. "Square bales," I asked?

"For quite a while we did some square and some round bales. The horse people like the smaller, square bales."

"Still doing the hay yourself?" I asked, suspecting the answer.

"Oh no, we lease the land out now. But I go out to the barn every day."

"100 acres. Who buys all those round bales?" I asked.

"We've had the same family buying all our hay for over 40 years. They have milk cows."

I finished up and brought the discharge instructions. "See your family doctor in two days to check for infection. Sutures come out in 10 to 12 days. You must be extremely careful when using a knife. It's easy to cut yourself."

"My wife," he replied unhappily, "She took my knife away. How can you go out to the barn without a pocketknife? Can you believe it?"

I listened attentively. In front of me was an elderly man, declining but trying to stay active. Just wanting to go out to his old barn and do a few chores. His wife was looking out for him. Driving and caring for him. She was right. It was clearly best for him not to be using any sharp instruments. I could see myself in his spot in 20 years.

"No, I can't."

Prophecy

I was starting a lecture for emergency medicine residents about practicing medicine. What does the word doctor mean? In our case it is a qualified practitioner of medicine. Did they know where the word doctor came from? It was derived from the Latin verb "docere" meaning to teach. I asked if they thought doctors could tell the future? No one answered. The young physicians looked at me like I was crazy. Could a physician be a prophet? Not a religious prophet, but an inspired teacher, or someone who can predict the future. I believe there are many reasons why physicians are held in high esteem. With our many years of education, training and experience we develop special knowledge and skill. In many situations we know what the future holds. We should use this insight.

How do you use your stethoscope? To hear lung sounds? Of course. But almost anyone can use that scope and hear some sounds inside the chest. Knowing what to do about it is what sets physicians apart. Patients aren't quite sure what's going on as we listen to the chest. When I see a young patient in the ER, no matter the chief complaint, I don't ask if they are a smoker. Usually it's obvious: the pack of cigarettes in their shirt pocket on the chair, the distinctive smell of smoke, the stain on their lips and fingers. I wait. When auscultating their lungs, I listen carefully, first in the front, on both sides. I frown a bit. Then I listen over the back, I frown some more. I ask them to take a deep breath and cough. I hear the tell-tale coarse rattle of chronic bronchitis.

221

Moving back in front of them, I take the stethoscope out of my ears and say, "You have smokers' lung. How much do you smoke?" The patients usually look astonished. I know what the future holds for the patient if they don't quit: shortness of breath, COPD, likely a heart attack, stroke, or lung cancer. I tell them, "You must quit as soon as possible. If you do, your risk of serious heart and lung disease diminishes tremendously."

I am not sure how effective this is, but it is important. Patients usually consider and attempt to quit smoking multiple times before they are successful. We need to help start them on this difficult journey. Many of our ER patients are coming to us at a time of crisis and danger. It is also an opportunity to begin a treatment program, to learn, and to change directions. We should take advantage of this opportunity.

———————————

Another example of using our knowledge about the future is when using the Killip Classification for patients presenting with a heart attack.

Class	Physical Examination	Mortality Rate
I	No signs of heart failure	5 to 10 %

II	Mild pulmonary congestion	10 to 25 %
III	Pulmonary edema	25 to 50 %
IV	Hypotension; cardiogenic shock	70 to 90 %

This was first published in 1967. (Ref. 4). Even today with all our interventions (thrombolytic agents, catheterization labs, coronary care units) it is still useful. Class IV patients still have over 50 % mortality. The classification is done completely at the bedside. It takes only a few moments. Check the ECG, take a brief history, and perform a focused physical exam. Start the appropriate medications, call the cardiologist, and notify the cath lab. Many Class IV patients require intubation, their prognosis is horrible.

I recommend telling the patient and family something like this: "You are having a dangerous heart attack; your heart is failing. We'll transfer you to the cardiac cath lab shortly. Your lungs are filling with fluid so we must intubate you now to protect your breathing. After that you won't be able to talk. While we prepare you have a minute or two to speak with your spouse / family." Believe me, they will understand it may be the last time they speak with their loved one.

Interesting Cases

By the mid 2010's our Novi ER had become a busy place. Our group employed numerous physicians and MLP's. Many were young women, similar in age to many of the nurses. If it wasn't busy, shift change became a social event. Happy chatter about families, social life, activities, (and whispered gossip). The close friendship and rapport were obvious, and staff morale improved. I was the physician director of the ER and considered the staff and my physician colleagues to be good friends, but I had to marvel over the improved comradery. Eight of the women began to vacation together in Mexico. When they returned tales would circulate through the ER about the "Party Girls." I would hear bits and pieces of the escapades but being almost a generation older I wasn't provided the intimate details. Many of the stories became legends. Most were embellishments; at least I hoped.

One morning I saw Ella (one of our NP's) as a patient in the ER. She was accompanied by her good friend, Dr. Stephanie Murphy, (one of my partners). They had returned from a vacation. Ella's complaint was dizziness. I wondered if this was from too much alcohol and partying.

"What are you doing here? Why did you have to come to the ER? Did you have too much fun?" I playfully asked.

Ella protested, "No, no. I suddenly started to feel bad."

"Ok, tell me what happened," I said. She explained that she had started feeling dizzy, lightheaded, nauseous, and vomited a few times. She felt tired, weak and had a small headache. "Sounds like you're hung over to me," I said.

"No, no. I hardly drank any alcohol. What concerns me is my speech is off, and I'm having trouble walking" Ella related.

"When was your last drink? I asked. "Over 24 hours ago."

I suddenly realized something wasn't right. Ella could get anxious at times. She had tremendous empathy and compassion for patients, always concerned they might have something serious. But she was not hypochondriacal. Speech problems and trouble walking aren't alcohol hangover symptoms. Those are alcohol intoxication symptoms. She didn't smell of alcohol. I snapped out of my "friend" mode and into my physician role.

"Start from the beginning and tell me the progression of symptoms again," I inquired.

She repeated her story. This time I listened more carefully. What I heard scared me. It sounded like Ella (in her mid-30's) was having a dangerous brainstem stroke. I performed a thorough neurological exam. Her speech was mildly slurred. Her coordination was off (ataxia), and her gait hesitant, wide based and off balanced.

"Ella, I think you might be having a stroke. We'll call the stroke alert, consult neurology, and get a CT and CTA (CT angiogram a CT study with IV contrast / dye which shows blood vessels)."

My partner Stephanie admitted they had briefly considered a stroke, but they didn't want to believe it. Brainstem strokes are uncommon (and like all strokes) rare under age 50. They can start with minimal symptoms that stop and start, then progressively worsen, many times causing major disability and death. Early in their course the diagnosis is often missed (as I almost had).

Ella's CT and CTA confirmed a brainstem stroke with blockage in the arterial blood supply. She was transferred to the Neuro ICU for consultation with Neurology and Neurosurgery. Her prognosis was guarded, and almost impossible to predict. Despite treatment Ella's symptoms worsened, then stabilized. Serious speech, balance and mobility problems persisted. Thank goodness she survived. Ella was discharged to an inpatient rehabilitation center. It would be a long road back towards normal and no certainty she could ever work again. Later, Ella underwent extended outpatient therapy. Slowly and gradually, she regained function.

This event reminded me of a mistake I'd made 35 years before. A childhood friend had called to ask about some unusual symptoms he was having: intermittent numbness and tingling, dizziness, and balance problems. They would wax and wane. It didn't sound like anything I could diagnose. He was worried it could be MS (Multiple Sclerosis). I considered it briefly. Then reassured him that MS was uncommon in men and not likely. I didn't want to believe it was a possibility. I was wrong. His symptoms continued to worsen, and he was diagnosed with RRMS (relapsing-remitting MS). Unfortunately, there were no effective treatments (at that time). Perhaps that episode helped me wake up and perform as a physician (not as a friend) and helped me consider and diagnose Ella's stroke.

I'd heard from her many friends that Ella had over the past year made significant improvements. One memorable day she walked into the physician workstation. There were long hugs and broad smiles all around.

She thanked me and wanted to ask a question, "I passed hospital credentialing (approval to work). Would I be her supervising physician when she returned to the ER?"

I had to bite my lip to hold back tears of joy, "Absolutely."

Fred was a 67-year-old man with a history of mental illness and narcolepsy (uncontrolled daytime sleepiness). His relatives found him hallucinating, hollering at people who weren't there. Fred was angry, sweating, pacing, and hyperventilating. The family convinced him to come to the ER and drove him to our facility. His past medical problems included hypertension, mild COPD, and arthritis. His medications included dextroamphetamine for narcolepsy.

The triage nurse brought him and his nephew immediately to our quiet room. Occasionally patients will respond to a calm non-stimulating environment. Not this time. Fred screamed constantly and became combative. He tried to strike our nurse and pushed his nephew away. This situation is fraught with danger: to the patient, family, bystanders, and medical staff. Restraining patients in this condition can lead to cardiac or respiratory arrest. Left untreated most patients worsen and injure themselves or others. Many medications have been studied. There was no clear most effective one. We would try Ketamine, a drug used for anesthesia in veterinary and human medicine. It produces a trance-like state: sedation and amnesia. Importantly, it can be given IM.

We assembled a team: four large male security guards, me and an RN with a syringe containing a large dose (350 mg) of Ketamine. Running in together each man grabbed one extremity. We were able to hold Fred briefly on the gurney. Without removing his clothes, the RN plunged the needle deep into his buttock and injected the medication. Fred didn't like it one bit. His strength was tremendous, and as soon as the injection was finished, we let him go and left the room.

Over 30 minutes he gradually calmed down enough so we were able to enter the room. His exam was unremarkable except for hyperventilation and VS: HR of 156, BP of 200 / 120 and RR of 30. We placed him on oxygen and HR monitors and sent off a slew of blood tests including ABG's (arterial blood gasses), drawn directly from the radial artery at the wrist. With observation over two hours his VSs gradually returned to normal. He was admitted for further treatment and likely adjustment of his medications.

The only significant laboratory abnormality was pH 6.88 (normal 7.40), and bicarb 6.6 with (normal 24). Fred was tremendously acidotic. That explained his hyperventilation. With Fred's exertion he produced a large amount of acid. In the body acid combines with bicarb and converts to water and carbon dioxide. The excess carbon dioxide is exhaled during ventilation. Repeat pH and bicarb two hours later were in the normal range. The severe acidosis may explain why some patients with agitated delirium have a cardiac arrest. The heart is a muscle, and muscles do not function well with severe acid around. One could easily have a lethal cardiac arrhythmia, or the heart muscle could suddenly become weak and fail to pump blood.

One month later EMS brought in a patient in full cardiac arrest. It was a young obese male patient who was caught shoplifting and was chased out of a supermarket. The security guard easily caught him and placed him on his stomach and kept his knee on the man's back. Police were called. They arrived within three minutes. They heard the man say, "I can't breathe, I can't breathe," and saw him become unresponsive. CPR was immediately started, and EMS called. They arrived shortly, continued CPR, and brought him to our ER a few miles away. The EMS crew were unable to intubate the patient, so performed BVM ventilation en route.

Upon arrival to our ER the patient was in full cardiac and respiratory arrest. I was able to intubate him. The computerized medical record revealed he had been to our facility in the past. His medical history included morbid obesity, and alcohol and cocaine addiction. His heart tracing was flatline. The ABG's revealed a horribly low pH of 6.78 (severe acidosis). The chance to restart the heart beating is about zero, but we followed ACLS guidelines. I asked the EMS crew what they found. They said a crowd had gathered. One lady said she had seen the whole thing.

When asked if she saw any fight or trauma she said, "There was a brief wrestling match. The security guard had his knee on the man's lower back." She didn't see any restraint, hog tying, or anything that looked like it would stop a man from breathing. The EMS crew said the bystanders seemed shocked that the man stopped breathing. After numerous rounds of medications, I "Called" the code and pronounced the young man dead.

I notified the medical examiner, and the body was transported for a full autopsy. I later reviewed the autopsy report. There was a small amount of cocaine detected. The conclusion was death due to positional asphyxia (suffocation). I think that was only partially correct. There certainly was more to it than that. For more than two decades there have been many reports of young men dying from restraints while in police custody. Many of the autopsies had no significant findings. The cause of death is often listed as positional asphyxia.

I believe many of these deaths are from severe acidosis leading to a lethal cardiac arrhythmia or sudden heart failure. Obese or out of shape patients quickly become acidotic with exertion. Think of how short of breath they would get by running a 100-yard dash. Stimulant medications (cocaine, amphetamines etc.) constrict arterioles and don't allow good perfusion (blood flow) through muscle tissue. Even small amounts of these drugs would cause rapid accumulation of acid in the muscle and blood stream with any exertion.

The normal response we have to acid in the body is to hyperventilate. The acid (H+) combines with bicarb (HCO3) and produces water (H2O) and carbon dioxide (CO2). The equation is: H+ plus HCO3 produces H2O and CO2. The excess carbon dioxide stimulates ventilation and is exhaled out through the lungs.

Anything that inhibits a patient's ability to breathe will significantly impede this process and allow excess CO2 and acid to accumulate. Many things can inhibit breathing in these situations: obesity, fatigue, any chest wall restraint, any abdominal pressure. These limit movement of the diaphragm. Abdominal pressure increases with lying on your stomach, and a knee or anything on your back. An acidotic patient unable to hyperventilate would complain of being unable to breathe. The next time you run a 100-yard dash think about how hard you are breathing (most of us must stop due to shortness of breath). Anything that inhibits your breathing would be extremely uncomfortable.

Lastly, it has been documented that even with immediate resuscitation (in these situations) outcomes are dismal. In other situations of cardiac arrhythmia or suffocation (hanging / drowning) immediate resuscitation can result in good outcomes. This discrepancy can be explained by severe acidosis. Even in a hospital setting, patients who develop a cardiac arrhythmia or sudden heart failure from severe acidosis are often unable to be resuscitated. A severely acidotic heart that stops is difficult to restart.

———————————————

It was 8 o'clock on a Saturday morning. In room 11 was a 27-year-old man with chest pain.

"Good morning, I'm Dr. Thomson, tell me about your chest pain."

He started hesitantly, "Well actually, I was having sex with my wife, when I got this burning sensation in my chest. The pain wasn't severe. It was pretty mild, but after a few minutes it didn't go away. So, we stopped."

There were no other symptoms. He'd had heartburn a few times in the past. There was no history of medical problems or family history of heart disease. He was a nonsmoker.

I kidded him, "Was that typical, having sex in the morning?"

He replied, "Well, my wife and I haven't had sex in quite a while. We had our first baby three weeks ago."

"Congratulations. Three weeks postpartum!" I exclaimed. "Aren't you supposed to wait four to six weeks?"

"Yes," he said sheepishly, "We couldn't wait."

"How's your baby doing,"

"Great," he replied. "That's why I came. I want to be extra careful."

I went through the exam, perfectly normal. His ECG, perfect as well. Chest X-ray was negative. Labs returned normal: the troponin (cardiac enzyme) was 0.030 (normal was less than 0.040). His HEART Score was 2 (out of 10 points). Zero to 3 points was low risk (less than a 2 percent chance of heart attack in the next month). If I followed the "Chest Pain Guidelines" he would be discharged to follow up with his primary care physician. However, a couple things about his history bothered me. He described his pain as "Pretty mild," but he had come in for evaluation. He must have been concerned. Also, I had no solid explanation for it. Heartburn was the most likely cause, but there is no way to prove the diagnosis in the ER.

"I would like to be cautious. Let's keep you here and watch you for 4 hours. We'll repeat the troponin. If that's normal you can safely go home to see your family doctor," I advised.

"No problem," he said.

Four hours later we repeated his ECG and troponin. The ECG was identical to the previous one, perfectly normal. The troponin was 0.038. This was still in the normal range, but it was minimally increased from the previous 0.030 level. Abnormal levels that are rising correlate well with heart damage. Rising levels in the normal range had not been found to be related to cardiac ischemia or any dangerous heart problems. I wasn't sure why, but I didn't like his presentation and troponin results.

"We should keep you overnight in our Observation unit. They will repeat your ECG and blood tests. Likely do a cardiac echo and stress test tomorrow morning." He agreed and was transferred down the hall to the Obs (Observation) Unit.

The next day I was working. I saw an EMS crew rushing through our ER. They were transferring a patient to the cardiac cath lab at our main hospital for an emergency procedure. It was the 27-year-old man from the day before.

"What happened?" I asked.

"Failed the stress test," he replied.

"Good luck," I called after him.

Exercise treadmill testing can reliably detect CAD (Coronary Artery Disease). But it is rare under age 35, almost unheard of under age 30. I called the cardiac stress lab. They said his cardiac echo looked fine. He began the stress test, walking on the treadmill for just a minute or two. Then, he suddenly developed burning substernal chest pain and his ECG showed marked changes with ST segment elevation. They immediately stopped the test, and his discomfort disappeared. He was being transferred for immediate cardiac catheterization.

Later that day I received a call from the cardiologist, "We found a large occlusion in the proximal LAD (an arterial lesion called the widow maker, a critical blockage in the largest coronary artery. Strongly associated with sudden death). We were able to dilate the artery and place a stent. The artery has good blood flow now. His prognosis is excellent. He's one of the youngest patients we've ever stented. Why did you decide to keep him for a stress test? You likely saved his life."

Maybe. The truth was, I'd almost sent him home. I think the 43-year-old man with chest pain that died after I'd sent him home so many years before, made the difference. That is what saved this young man's life.

Epilogue

I completed my last two shifts in April of 2018. The majority of my 36-year career was spent in the ER in Novi. During the last 10 years I worked two to four shifts a month in the ER in Jackson. Caring for patients is a serious undertaking. I knew at times I could get emotional, so I was concerned about my last shift. I wanted to ensure I would concentrate on properly caring for each patient. I scheduled my second to last shift in Novi, and the very last one in Jackson.

On my last day at the Novi ER the medical care of patients was routine. Many of the staff stopped by to give me a hug and offer congratulations. They knew this day was coming. Some were quite tearful, of course I would miss them too. Surprisingly my eyes remained dry, even when walking out. I was happy and content, thankful for tremendous good fortune that had befallen me. I had put my heart and soul into practicing medicine. I was only a little sad. I reached my destination, the finish of a challenging and rewarding journey.

My last shift in Jackson went smoothly. The staff knew it was my final day. I was scheduled until midnight and finished just after 1 AM. I made extra sure there were no loose ends regarding my patients. I gave a final report. My career in Emergency Medicine: the long days and fatiguing nights, the unforeseen events, the highs and lows, the joyful triumphs and horrible tragedies, had ended.

My newest partner Dr. Jake Sinkoff quietly gave me a present: a small fly box with a few flies. He knew about my passion for catching small brook trout on dry flies.

I had revealed to him a secret location in Michigan's Upper Peninsula where every sunny August afternoon the trout rise to the surface chasing ants and grasshoppers. It's a shallow, intricate, remote stream. Crystal clear water gurgles softly as it rushes back and forth between overhanging tag alders and fallen logs.

I hadn't told him about the best place, a mile and half further downstream. It's an extended wade through "spreads" and cedar swamp. The brook trout are wary. If you sneak along slowly, they rise freely to dry flies. There are no signs of civilization, it is true wilderness. I often fish there alone. The stream continues through even more impenetrable cedar swamp. I'm not sure anyone has ever fished there. If I have enough courage, that may be my next adventure.

Lessons

Nothing much good happens after midnight. Best to be at home sleeping.

I learn more while listening than I do while talking. When everyone agrees with me and my opinion, I feel comfortable. When someone disagrees with me, I learn more. It takes courage to express a different or minority opinion. I need to be open to them.

Verbal communication is direct and fast. Nonverbal communication (appearance, dress, eye contact, facial expression, tone of voice, body language, gestures, posture, position, touch) is at least as important and conveys valuable information (intentions, needs, emotions, attitudes). Skills in both are required by emergency physicians. Especially during the initial patient encounter, (to establish rapport) and during the final discussion (when summarizing what has happened and describing what the future may hold).

Find a good mentor. They will share their knowledge and expertise. Your learning curve, confidence and problem-solving skills will accelerate tremendously.

Be cautious when someone says, "I'm not lying to you," they quite often just did.

Concussions and head injuries cause brain damage. The research is unequivocal. We need to protect our brain. Boxing and any sport or activity that has a goal of injuring the head (brain) should be changed or abandoned. No state or country should sanction them.

Outdoor walks and activities are tremendously healthy for body and mind; for everyone; the young and the old.

I've been told I have a biased opinion. Of course I do. I worked in the ER for 36 years.

"Make everyone on your team better." What a fantastic attitude to have; in sports and in life. Winning is overrated. To actively participate is the most important thing.

"If I have seen further it is by standing on the shoulders of giants." In a letter from Isaac Newton (1642 - 1727) to Robert Hooke; dated 1675. Physicians and patients are in debt to all scientists who contributed to the development and practice of medicine.

References

1. Jameson, J. L., & Loscalzo, J. (1976). Harrison's Principles of Internal Medicine (3rd edition). New York: McGraw Hill Education.

2. Silen, W. (1980). Cope's Early Diagnosis of the Acute Abdomen (15th edition). New York: Oxford University Press.

3. Stephan Rieeel, MD, PhD. Edward Jenner and the history of smallpox and vaccination. Baylor Univ Med Cent Proceedings, 18:1, Jan 2005, pp 21-25.

4. Killip T, Kimball JT. Treatment of myocardial infarction in a coronary care unit. A two-year experience with 250 patients. Am J Cardiol, 20:4, Oct 1967, pp 457-64.

5. Mark Thomson, MD. Guns and Humans. Unpublished Editorial. April 2002.

Abbreviations

AAA:	Abdominal Aortic Aneurysm
ABEM:	American Board of Emergency Medicine
ABG's:	Arterial Blood Gasses
ABMS:	American Board of Medical Specialties
ACLS:	Advanced Cardiac Life Support
AFM:	Acute Flaccid Myelitis
AIDS:	Autoimmune Deficiency Syndrome
AMI:	Acute Myocardial Infarction / Heart Attack
AP:	Anterior Posterior / Front Back
APGAR:	Appearance, Pulse, Grimace, Activity, Respiration
ASAP:	As Soon As Possible
BC:	Board Certified
BP:	Blood Pressure
BPD:	BronchoPulmonary Dysplasia
BVM:	Bag, Valve, Mask
CAD:	Coronary Artery Disease
Cath:	Catheterization

CC:	Chief Complaint
CCU:	Coronary Care Unit
CHF:	Congestive Heart Failure
CO2:	Carbon Dioxide
COPD:	Chronic Obstructive Pulm Disease (Smokers Lung)
CPR:	CardioPulm Resuscitation (Chest Compressions)
CSF:	CerebroSpinal Fluid
CT:	Computerized Tomography
CTA:	CT Angiography
CXR:	Chest X ray
CVA:	Cerebral Vascular Accident / Stroke
DHHS:	Department of Health and Human Services
DKA:	Diabetic KetoAcidosis
DNR:	Do Not Resuscitate
DO:	Doctor of Osteopathic Medicine
DTR:	Deep Tendon Reflexes
DT's	Delirium Tremens
ECG:	Electrocardiogram

ED: Emergency Department

EM: Emergency Medicine

EMS: Emergency Medical Service / Ambulance

EMT: Emergency Medical Technician

EMTALA: Emergency Medical Treatment and Labor Act

ENT: Ear, Nose and Throat

EOM: Extra Ocular Movements

ER: Emergency Room

ET: Endotracheal

ETA: Estimated Time of Arrival

Fam Hx: Family History

FP: Family Practice

GB: Gallbladder

GCS: Glascow Coma Scale

GI: Gastrointestinal

GPA: Grade Point Average

GS: General Surgery

HA: Headache

HEART:	Heart Score: Heart, ECG, Age, Risk, Troponin
Hem / Onc	Hematology / Oncology
HIV:	Human Immunodeficiency Virus
HR:	Heart Rate
ICD:	Implantable Cardioverter Defibrillator
ICU:	Intensive Care Unit
IM:	Internal Medicine
IM:	Intramuscular
IO:	Interosseous
INR:	Blood Test for Amount of Blood Thinner
IV:	Intravenous Line
IVP:	Intravenous Push
JVD:	Jugular (neck) Venous Distention
L:	Lumbar
LAD:	Left Anterior Descending
LKN:	Last Known Normal
LMP:	Last Menstrual Period
LOC:	Level Of Consciousness

LP:	Lumbar Puncture
ME:	Medical Examiner
Med Rec:	Medical Records
MERS:	Middle Eastern Respiratory Syndrome
MLP:	Midlevel Provider / NP or PA
MRI:	Magnetic Resonance Imaging
MS:	Multiple Sclerosis
MVA:	Motor Vehicle Accident
NC:	Nasal Cannula
NP:	Nurse Practitioner
NS:	Normal Saline
NSR:	Normal Sinus Rhythm
NTG:	Nitroglycerin
OBs	Observation Unit
OB / GYN:	Obstetrics / Gynecology
OR:	Operating Room
Ox:	Oxygen
PA:	Physician Assistant

PALS:	Pediatric Advanced Life Support
PCN:	Penicillin
PCP:	Primary Care Physician
PCR:	Polymerase Chain Reactiont for Bacteria / Virus
PE:	Pulmonary Embolism
PEEP:	Peak End Expiratory Pressure
PFO:	Patent Foramen Ovale
PGY:	Post Graduate Year I, II, III
PMHx:	Past Medical History
pOx:	Pulse Oxygen - Percent Oxygen
PPE:	Personal Protective Equipment
QT:	An Interval on the ECG
RBC's:	Red Blood Cells
Ref:	Reference
ROM:	Range of Motion
ROS:	Review Of Symptoms
RR:	Respiratory Rate
RRMS:	Relapsing Remitting Multiple Sclerosis

RSI:	Rapid Sequence Intubation
RSV:	Respiratory Syncytial Virus
RT:	Respiratory Therapist
RUQ:	Right Upper Quadrant, LUQ; RLQ; LLQ
RV:	Right Ventricle
Rx:	Prescription
SARS:	Severe Acute Respiratory Syndrome
SBO:	Small Bowel Obstruction
SL:	Sublingual
SLE:	Systemic Lupus Erythematosus
SOB:	Shortness of Breath
ST:	A Segment on the ECG
STAT:	Immediately
TIA:	Transient Ischemic Attack
TMJ:	TemporoMandibular Joint
UA:	Urine Analysis
UC:	Urgent Care
URI:	Upper Respiratory Illness / cold

US: Ultrasound

UTI: Urinary Tract Infection

V Fib: Ventricular Fibrillation. A lethal arrhythmia

VS   Vital Signs

V Tach: Ventricular Tachycardia.

WBC: White Blood Cell

Guns and Humans

Every health care provider who has worked in an ER anywhere in the United States is familiar with victims of interpersonal violence. Similar to police officers we often see patients due to events when people are at their worst. I tried to have faith in the inherent goodness of my fellow man but nearly every week I was confronted with evidence to the contrary. Most people most of the time are calm, reasonable, considerate, and rational. However, during stressful moments humans are prone to quick reactions, anger, and uncontrolled behavior. Brief episodes of hostility, rage and violence can occur, resulting in traumatic injuries and death. Too often the most lethal weapon available is used.

Perpetrators use hands, feet, and mouth as weapons. Typical injuries are bruises, fractures, head injuries, bite wounds and strangulations. Some deaths occur. If objects such as belts, clubs or bats are used the injuries are similar in pattern but more severe. Due to the increased forces applied more deaths occur. If a knife is used the incidence of serious injury or death increases further. Fortunately, it is relatively difficult to injure multiple people during one incident with a knife.

If a gun is used, the likelihood of major injury and death increases immensely. Unfortunately, it is easy to injure or kill multiple people during one incident with a gun. Add in the ready availability of high-volume ammunition clips and the damage is exponentially magnified. I predict when guns are readily available many episodes of catastrophic injuries and multiple deaths will result. That is wrong. The carnage from gun violence is already occurring. The United States has more guns and more gun violence than any country in the world. The ratio of gun ownership to incidence of gun violence correlates well across every country. Americans have 5 percent of the world's population. We have 42 percent of privately owned firearms.

Violent behavior by humans has been documented throughout recorded human history. Despite civilization, societal customs, religion, laws, regulations, etc violence continues unabated. The only predictive characteristic of perpetrators of gun violence is that they are more likely to be men. Of course, there are women perpetrators too. A history of mental illness is uncommon.

It is easier to buy a gun then to obtain a driver's license.

Buying a gun for personal protection is the top reason for owning a firearm. This is a misconception. Owning a gun significantly **increases** the risk of death from accidents, suicide, and domestic violence. These events most often involve family members. Criminal homicides are thirty five times more likely than a justifiable homicide from defensive gun use. Buying a gun markedly decreases your safety (and your families).

The Second Amendment to the US Constitution was ratified on December 15, 1791. The only firearms readily available were muskets and flintlock pistols. I am sure our forefathers had not considered powerful semi and fully automatic weapons with large capacity ammunition clips. The Constitution is meant to be a flexible document. That is why our forefathers included a process for Amendments. Large capacity ammunition clips are weapons of war. They should be outlawed.

All sides in the gun control argument (manufacturers, owners, and non-owners) should work together to end gun violence.

I tire of hearing a regulation is an attack on our freedom. Wearing a seatbelt and driving less than 90 miles an hour on the highway impacts your freedom. Both are common sense regulations to ensure your own and other people's safety.

There should be mandatory training and licensing for gun owners (similar to drivers). Require safe and secure gun storage. This would help minimize the horrible tragedies among children and suicidal patients. Support CVI (Community Violence Intervention) programs, they have been effective in reducing gun violence. Expand gun violence research. Improve the National Crime Information Center database. Require background checks on all gun sales.

Guns and humans don't mix. When they do, serious injury and death follow. Alcohol is a dangerous drug. It causes serious medical illness and is a significant contributor to sudden death: overdoses, fights, gun violence, drunk driving, etc.

I recall a picture in Life magazine years ago, an advertisement painted on the side of a gasoline station convenience store. It read: **"Liquor Guns Ammunition Picnic Supplies."** What could possibly go wrong? (Ref. 5).

www.ingramcontent.com/pod-product-compliance
Lightning Source LLC
Chambersburg PA
CBHW021921190326
41519CB00009B/869